Biomarkers and Biosensors for Cervical Cancer Diagnosis

John Bosco Balaguru Rayappan •
Jung Heon Lee
Editors

Biomarkers and Biosensors for Cervical Cancer Diagnosis

Springer

Editors
John Bosco Balaguru Rayappan
Centre for Nanotechnology & Advanced Biomaterials (CeNTAB), School of Electrical and Electronics Engineering
SASTRA Deemed University
Thanjavur, Tamil Nadu, India

Jung Heon Lee
School of Advanced Materials Science and Engineering, Research Center for Advanced Materials Technology, Biomedical Institute for Convergence at SKKU (BICS)
Sungkyunkwan University (SKKU)
Suwon, Republic of Korea

ISBN 978-981-16-2585-5 ISBN 978-981-16-2586-2 (eBook)
https://doi.org/10.1007/978-981-16-2586-2

This Springer imprint is published by the registered company Springer Nature Singapore Pte Ltd.
The registered company address is: 152 Beach Road, #21-01/04 Gateway East, Singapore 189721, Singapore

Acknowledgments

The editors are grateful to the Ministry of Human Resource Development, Government of India for funding the project titled "Affordable Colorimetric and Electrochemical Biosensors for the Early-Stage Detection of Cervical Cancer" through Scheme for Promotion of Academic and Research Collaboration (SPARC) "SPARC/2018-2019/P402/SL." We also acknowledge the support received from the National Research Foundation (NRF) of Korea for the Basic Science Research Program funded by the Ministry of Education (NRF-2019R1A6A1A03033215). We are grateful to SASTRA Deemed University, Thanjavur, India and Sungkyunkwan University (SKKU), South Korea for providing infrastructural support. We would like to express our heartfelt gratitude to the contributing authors, who assisted us in the development of this book. We would also like to express our gratitude to Dr. Bhavik Sawhney, Editor-Biomedicine, Springer Nature for his feedback, guidance, and support in finalizing this book.

Contents

About the Editors

John Bosco Balaguru Rayappan is a Professor and Dean-Sponsored Research at SASTRA Deemed University, Thanjavur, Tamil Nadu, India. Presently, he is heading the Nanosensors Laboratory at SASTRA through research grants obtained from DST, New Delhi, DRDO, New Delhi, DBT, New Delhi and SASTRA Deemed University. His research interests are across diverse fields of Lattice Dynamics, Nanosensors, Biosensors, Embedded System and IoT. He has published more than 310 research articles in these fields and filed 7 patents including one US patent. He is editorial board member and reviewer for several journals and has 25 years of teaching experience.

Jung Heon Lee is an Associate Professor in the School of Advanced Materials Science and Engineering at Sungkyunkwan University (SKKU). He is also affiliated with Biomedical Institute for Convergence at SKKU (BICS), the Institute of Quantum Biophysics (IQB), and the Research Center for Advanced Materials Technology at SKKU. Prof. Lee is leading the Biological and Nanoscale Materials Laboratory at SKKU, where he is focused on developing nanoscale materials or devices which can be applied to diverse levels of biological systems for diagnostics or therapeutics. He is also investigating opportunities to adapt programmable and readily modifiable properties of biomolecules in the fabrication of smart materials or advanced nanoscale devices. He has also published more than 85 research articles in peer-reviewed international journals and filed 50 patents, including 7 US patents and 5 PCT patents.

An Introduction to Cancer Biomarkers

1

Muthaiyan Lakshmanakumar, Arockia Jayalatha JBB, and
Noel Nesakumar

Abstract

Cancer is the abnormal growth of cells due to the accumulation of changes in the genetic program that regulates the proliferation, growth and survival of cells. The impact of cancer on society is huge and hence, rapid, efficient and reliable detection is deemed essential in cancer management since it can lead to successful medical strategies, reduce treatment expenses and dramatically improve patient outcomes and survival rate. In this context, the barriers to cancer diagnosis and various approaches, including ultrasound, thermography, X-ray, tissue biopsy and optical techniques, pertaining to cancer detection are elucidated in this book chapter, with a special focus on how analytical techniques help clinicians detect cancers at an early stage. The merits and demerits of these analytical techniques for detecting cancers are also discussed in this book chapter. Finally, advances in

M. Lakshmanakumar
Centre for Nanotechnology and Advanced Biomaterials (CeNTAB), SASTRA Deemed University, Thanjavur, Tamil Nadu, India

School of Electrical and Electronics Engineering, SASTRA Deemed University, Thanjavur, Tamil Nadu, India

A. J. JBB
School of Electrical and Electronics Engineering, SASTRA Deemed University, Thanjavur, Tamil Nadu, India

N. Nesakumar (✉)
Centre for Nanotechnology and Advanced Biomaterials (CeNTAB), SASTRA Deemed University, Thanjavur, Tamil Nadu, India

School of Chemical and Biotechnology, SASTRA Deemed University, Thanjavur, Tamil Nadu, India
e-mail: noel@scbt.sastra.edu

J. B. B. Rayappan, J. H. Lee (eds.), *Biomarkers and Biosensors for Cervical Cancer Diagnosis*, https://doi.org/10.1007/978-981-16-2586-2_1

biotechnology science that have contributed to the development of biosensors for cancer detection are outlined.

Keywords

Cervical cancer · HPV · DNA · Cancer diagnosis · X-ray

1.1 Introduction

Cancer is the abnormal growth of cells due to the accumulation of mutations in the genetic program that regulates the proliferation, growth and survival of cells [1, 2]. When cancer metastasizes, the tumour starts spreading beyond the primary site and rapidly spreads throughout the body to several other organs, making it untreatable. There are more than 200 different types of cancer, including leukaemia, colon, skin, hematologic, ovarian, breast, prostate lung cancer and more. Also, a few cancers such as cervical and stomach cancer are directly linked to viral and bacterial infections, respectively [3, 4].

Cancer is considered as the second most common cause of death worldwide. The World Health Organization (WHO) report indicates that the number of cancer-related deaths in 2014 was nearly 1.3 million in the European Union and in 2015, around 8.8 million people worldwide died of cancer. In the year 2014, the average mortality rate in the European Union was almost 261.5 per 100,000 people, which was significantly lower than the mortality rate for heart diseases; however, higher than the average mortality rate for several other causes of death. It is also predicted that during the lifetime of men and women, 38.4% of men and women worldwide will be diagnosed with cancer, according to the National Institutes of Health. About 1.1 crore people are expected to develop cancer each year and it is predicted that 1.6 crore people will be diagnosed with cancer by 2020 [5, 6].

The impact of cancer on society is huge and hence rapid, efficient and reliable detection is deemed essential in cancer management since it can lead to successful medical strategies, reduce treatment expenses and dramatically improve patient outcomes and survival rate. Cancer is an extremely heterogeneous disease that presents a wide variety of genetic and morphological variations that in turn shapes its prognosis in clinical practice. In particular, cancers develop gradually over time in response to specific exogenous and/or endogenous stimuli. Cancer can indeed be described as a breakdown in the communication network of cells. The genetic changes lead to modified proteins which induce stimuli that interact with normal cellular pathways. Early diagnosis of cancer is a political and public concern and primary care is the preferred framework for this to happen. Advancements in the early diagnosis of cancer have led to a need for improved cancer screening tests, preferably those that can be used in primary care. Nevertheless, continuous and extensive work in the development of new biomarkers and other assessments has had a positive impact on the prognosis and evaluation of patients previously diagnosed with the disease. In particular, there are few advantages to enhance the accuracy and promptness of cancer diagnosis in cancer patients who typically have symptoms. A broad variety of screening tests could be beneficial. A wide variety of stakeholders, including industry, investors, health care professionals, policymakers and customers, have recognized this great challenge to improve the accurate diagnosis of cancer [7, 8].

Cervical cancer, induced by the exponential proliferation of cells in the cervix, is one of the deadliest illnesses that requires extensive research in the field of biosensor for ultra-low detection of biomarkers specific to cervical cancer. The human papillomavirus (HPV) induces cervical cancer, which is a common sexually transmitted disease that affects the female reproductive system. Cervical cancer has become the leading cause of death after breast cancer, which has affected the socialization of the working environment of women. With operational excellence in diagnostic techniques and vaccination strategies in developed countries, the rapid recognition of early stage cervical cancer in women living in resource-limited settings with adequate medication has become a crucial requirement. At first glance, HPV may appear to be a genetically engineered cancer-causing machine, but, of the 150 HPV genotypes identified, only a few are high risk or oncogenic. Although in many HPV-infected patients the virus is rapidly removed through their own immune response, some people could be asymptomatic as the virus remains in an inactive state, and several other infected individuals may develop recurrent infections [9, 10]. Several attributes, including localization, spread, size and lesion type, determine the degree of HPV infection and assist clinicians to choose the correct treatment. Cervical cancer is usually curable if diagnosed and treated early, but in later stages, the cancer spreads throughout the body to the remaining part of the abdominal walls, rectum, bladder and uterus and eventually enters the pelvic lymphatic system, affecting other organ systems and resulting in death. Therefore, it is highly desirable to diagnose cancer at an early stage and to plan for effective drugs. Traditional histological techniques have poor accuracy and efficacy in the early detection of cancer, although they are time intensive. It is therefore essential to develop innovative tools for the rapid recognition of specific biomarkers and for monitoring therapeutic responses. Electrochemical techniques explore innovative ways to operate quickly and selectively, as cells immobilized on the surface of the electrode can generate electrochemical signals that can be beneficial in the design and fabrication of effective biosensors. The oxidation process and the ion changes that take place owing to distinct cellular functions result in the generation and transfer of electrons at the surface of living cells, and therefore, the living cell is considered to be an electrochemical system. Conversely, there are also many sensors available in the market to recognize the types of HPV. In particular, CLART®human papillomavirus 2, clinical arrays®HPV, INNO-LiPA, PapilloCheck®, linear array®, digene HC2 high-risk HPV DNA and COBAS®4800 are the main commercially exploited biosensors that provide enhanced sensitivity for ultra-low detection of pre-cancerous lesions and HPVs in human blood serum samples. Besides that, the techniques listed have shortcomings, including sophisticated equipment, the need for trained personnel, high response time and consumption of expensive reagent [11–13]. Therefore, despite the various drawbacks of established detection techniques, it is essential to design and develop an effective advanced analytical tool for the recognition of HPV with high selectivity and improved sensitivity.

The obstacle in the diagnosis and monitoring of cancer is to identify these proteins, renegade genes as well as other biochemical compounds, including cancer-related biomarkers at a very initial stage. Healthcare professionals had recognized cancer according to its pathology before molecular detection was feasible, which is associated with its appearance under the microscope of tissue sections of the patient [14–16]. Early detection and selective drugs are the existing practical strategies that impact the lives and health of cancer sufferers. Conversely, prior to the actual onset of the disease, rapid, inexpensive and robust diagnosis of cancer markers in human blood and other such bioavailable fluids makes it possible to study the development of tumour. Conversely, significant advancements with an in-depth understanding of the growth of tumour at the cellular, molecular and genetic levels help to develop accurate diagnostic methods to identify cancer markers at the molecular level. Substantial developments have been achieved in the identification of human tumours over the past decade [17–19]. Because of the expertise gained from emerging fields including molecular imaging, metabolomics, proteomics and genomics, cancer cells can now be characterized at genetic and molecular levels via employing advanced molecular tools, including protein and gene chips, mass spectroscopy and positron emission tomography. Molecular detection can assess how well these proteins and genes communicate through patterns of activity within the cell [20–23]. Such altered expression patterns in various kinds of cancer cells or "molecular fingerprints" enhance the potential for doctors to diagnose cancer. Molecular changes in cancer cells can be analysed by examining the sequence and genetic information of deoxyribonucleic acid (DNA) and the levels of metabolic products and proteins. The gene expression patterns and the number of copies of DNA, in particular, are key characteristics for the identification of cancer cells. The advances in DNA array technology have enabled reliable and quantifiable measurements of alterations in gene expression and chromosomal gains in human tumours [24, 25]. The individual tumour cell can be characterized by unique molecular specifics in conjunction with specific gene sequencing aimed at looking for point mutations. Over the past few years, recognizing single nucleotide-polymorphism-based genotyping to identify alleles associated with a greater risk of acquiring several diseases, including cancer, diabetes or other illnesses, has also been gaining popularity and significance among doctors and the wider community. These emerging innovations and the level of knowledge of molecular signatures will improve the ability to destabilize disease progression by monitoring, controlling and catalysing progress toward the use of targeted cancer therapies. In addition to the use of specific body fluids and tissue for in vitro characterization of biomolecules as cancer biomarkers, molecular imaging approaches concentrated primarily on positron emission tomography and magnetic resonance imaging [26–28].

Usually, understanding tumour's molecular environments is imperative for guiding and offering better treatment options in clinical settings. Tissue biopsies are the popularly adopted method of obtaining specific tumour molecular information and are required to identify its nature, including screening, expression of mutations in genes and the type of cancer. Nevertheless, it is full of issues, including the need for invasive surgical extraction, which may induce pain and discomfort in individuals. The clinical strategies associated with tissue biopsy involve many health risks and the likelihood of medical complications [29–31]. In addition, some tumours are inaccessible in certain anatomical sites, which are not suitable for a biopsy, and, in certain instances, their extraction may increase the risk of metastatic lesions. Often, the amount of tissue sample collected is insufficient for all diagnostic tests and the action must be carried out once again, which becomes necessary even otherwise if the tumour is not homogeneous [32–34]. In addition, the solid biopsy techniques are time consuming in terms of analysis, entails huge expenses and needs an operating theatre. Although biopsies from different metastatic sites can be performed at the same time, initiation of treatment may be delayed due to examination of the samples. In addition, tumour development desperately needs to be examined at different intervals for cost-effective treatment of the illness, so that solid biopsies can no longer be considered as highly invasive [35–37]. Typically, optical approaches are employed; yet, they do not render significant information about tumour. Radiology is often used routinely, but high levels of radiation can pose a health risk to the patient. Conversely, magnetic resonance imaging (MRI), a non-radiation method, is regarded as unreliable and unsuitable for the detection of minimal residual disease. In addition, safety is a concern, for example, in patients with comorbid conditions. Such approaches are also clinically impracticable and cannot cover the tumour's spatial and temporal heterogeneity [38–40].

X-ray allows clinicians to examine cancer in various parts of the body, including kidney, stomach and bones. Contrast analyses may need further planning in advance and can induce some pain and health risks based on the type of contrast materials employed. Typically, chest X-ray is the first assessment tool employed to detect lung cancer. Majority of lung tumours are present as a greyish white cloud on X-rays [41–43]. Chest X-rays, however, do not provide an appropriate diagnosis because they cannot differentiate between other conditions and cancer, including a lung abscess. Moreover, it produces harmful radiations which can pave the way for the possibility of cancer. In contrast, certain cytology assessments, including the Pap test, are being used primarily for screening, whereas others recognize cancers reliably. A diagnostic procedure is most often used when a screening test is positive [44–46].

Thermography, a non-invasive diagnostic tool, is a painless, rapid and cost-effective technique used to measure the temperature of the skin surface in a non-contact mode. Thermography is commonly used in the diagnosis of cancer and has been the focus of numerous biomedical researches in recent decades. Few thermography-based cancer diagnosis findings indicate that the venous blood entering the cancer location is always hotter than its arterial supply. Nevertheless, thermograms alone will not suffice to make an effective clinical diagnosis for healthcare professionals. The integration of statistical tools, including non-linear regression methods and artificial neural networks, is strongly recommended to accurately assess the thermogram [47, 48].

Ultrasound has played an important role in detecting cancer as a standard medical imaging method. The general characteristics that the ultrasound diagnosis of cancer shed light on are contours, internal structure, orientation and morphology of lesions, which produce a high diagnostic accuracy [49–51]. However, in the case of greater depth, a lower frequency is needed to obtain optimal images and, therefore, an image of lower resolution is obtained. Very accurate detection of cancer is important to provide the best therapeutic effectiveness. While endoscopy with multiple biopsies is a prerequisite for successful cancer diagnosis, endoscopic ultrasound and positron emission tomography-computed scanning (PET-CT) are considered appropriate techniques for accurate cancer diagnosis. PET-CT scans are a kind of assessment that generates 3-dimensional images of the body's interior. Such clinical tests are employed to assess distant, local and regional distribution [52–54]. The imaging techniques used to diagnose cancer correctly and completely are analogous; the use of a single tool is associated with negative effects and inadequate for a proper diagnosis.

Conversely, specific methods of cancer treatment, which include radiation therapy, surgery and chemotherapy, are typically associated with early differentiation of cancer cells. Hence, diagnosis of cancer is important for the early characterization of an effective cancer treatment [55–57]. The use of bio-sensing devices could be crucial in the early diagnosis of cancer, especially in cancer patients who are usually diagnosed at later stages and react negatively to treatment, thus leading to improvements in the quality of lifestyle in patients.

Although technological advances are producing a progressive series of new diagnostic tests that include artificial intelligence algorithms, imaging tools, sensors and biomarkers, the overwhelming majority of early-stage cancer detection tests fail since they do not work properly in populations with low susceptibility. In addition to this, a test performed in a population with higher susceptibility to the disease would generally be less sensitive when performed in a population with a lower prevalence of the disease. This results in an increase in false positive tests [58–60]. Therefore, difficulties in assessing cancer, as well as other low-prevalence conditions, involve overdiagnosis and overinvestigation, deciding on the standard criterion to be used to assess the efficacy of the tests and related outcomes.

The prospect of cancer management is believed to be highly dependent on the use of biomarkers that direct clinicians at every stage of disease management. Tumour biomarkers are biochemical compounds associated with the growth of malignant tumours in body tissue, urine or blood [61–63]. Normally, they are produced directly by tumour tissue or embryonic tissue. Biomarkers represent variations in protein expression that are strongly associated with the advancement of a disease or its therapy response and can be assessed in blood or tissues. Biomarkers can therefore be hormones or specific cells, enzymes or gene products, genes or molecules [64–66]. Biomarkers associated with cancer could be used in different stages to reliably diagnose and treat the disease. These can be effective in predicting different aspects during the onset of disease, which include early diagnosis, prediction of outcomes and identification of recurrence of disease. Notably, with the emergence of several new therapeutic agents, suitable biomarkers can be employed to assess which tumours will respond to certain therapies in order to evaluate the impact of drug resistance [67–69].

Over the past decade, advances in biotechnological research have facilitated the development of biosensors. Typically, biosensors are compact analytical systems containing at least one biomolecule. The integration of miniaturized electrodes with the immobilized biomolecule capable of detecting cancer biomarkers with high sensitivity and specificity are the desired attributes of a biosensor, which makes it suitable for rapid clinical analysis. Materials structure at the nanoscale including nanocomposites, nanofibers, nanotubes and nanoparticles has been employed to aid performance of these sensors. These nanoscale materials are substantially important for providing improved interfacial modification alternatives to increase the sensitivity of biosensors and improve the analytical signal [70–72]. The challenges related to the design of these miniaturized bio-sensing devices depend on the need to retain the biological activity of the immobilized biomolecules and the electron shuttling capability of nanomaterials. Over the past decade, a plethora of research papers on the use of biosensors in cancer monitoring and detection have been published which provide a detailed analysis of the physical–chemical properties of both constituents.

1.1.1 Epidemiology and Aetiology of Cervical Cancer

Cancer has a huge influence on society in the USA and around the world. Statistics on cancer explain what occurs in large numbers of people and provide insight into how cancer affects society [73]. Statistics give us information on the number of people who end up dying from cancer each year. Cancer statistics also show how many individuals are diagnosed with cancer each year. In addition, it also points out the mean age at diagnosis and the number of individuals presently living after a cancer diagnosis [74]. They also give us information about disparities between agc, geographical location, sex, ethnic/racial groups and other categories. Although statistical results are generally not directly relevant to individual patients, they are important for researchers, health professionals, policymakers and governments to recognize the effect of cancer on the population and establish approaches to manage the difficulties that cancer brings to society at large. In addition, statistical analysis is significant to assess the progress of cancer control and management efforts [74].

Cancer is the world's second-largest cause of mortality. Cancer is expected to cause 960,000 deaths in 2018. Approximately one in six deaths worldwide is due to cancer. Especially, in low- and middle-income countries, nearly 70% of cancer deaths occur. Approximately, one-third of cancer deaths are attributed to the five dietary and major lifestyle risks: alcohol consumption, tobacco usage, lack of exercise, poor consumption of vegetables and fruits and high mass index. Among the major lifestyle risks, smoking is the most significant cause of cancer and is accountable for about 22% of deaths due to cancer. Cancer that causes infections, including human papillomavirus and hepatitis, accounts for up to 25% of cancer deaths in middle- and low-income countries [74]. Statistical studies of cancer deaths suggest that late detection and mistreatment are the main reasons for the increasing incidence of cancer deaths in low- and middle-income countries. In 2017, the public sector had limited access to pathology services in 26% of low-income countries. Treatment services are offered to more than 90% of people diagnosed with cancer in high-income countries, while treatment services are provided to less than 30% of people diagnosed with cancer in low-income countries [65].

The economic implications of cancer are considerable, not only for cancer patients and also for society in general. According to the report of Agency for Healthcare Research and Quality (AHRQ), an estimate of $80.2 billion has been allocated for healthcare costs in the USA [2]. Of which, 52% of the total cost was allocated to hospitalized patients and 38% of the total cost was reserved for inpatient hospital stays. In contrast, the average monthly expenses required to receive adequate cancer treatment is high in low- and middle-income countries. According to statistics collected from World Bank in 2013, it has been found that only 13.7% of health expenditure is covered in high-income countries, 33.3% in upper-middle income countries, 52.8% in lower-middle income countries and 48.1% in low-income countries.

As of January 1, 2019, nearly 16.9 million people living in the USA with a history of cancer were alive; many of them were diagnosed several years ago and did not have new evidence of cancer. In the USA, over 1.8 million new cancer cases are expected to be diagnosed by 2020 [57, 58]. This assessment does not consider non-invasive cancer of any location, except the urinary bladder. It is projected that around 600,000 Americans will die of cancer by 2020. According to the statistical report on cancer incidence in the USA, the most common cancers identified in 2018 are liver cancer, thyroid cancer, pancreatic cancer, leukaemia, endometrial cancer, kidney and renal pelvis cancer, non-Hodgkin lymphoma, bladder cancer, melanoma of the skin, colon and rectum cancer, prostate cancer, lung and bronchus cancer and breast cancer [43–45].

Cancer mortality rates are the best indicator of advancement against the disease as screening methods impact them less than new cancer diagnoses and overall survival. In 2018, the mortality of cancer is greater among men than among women. While examining groups based on sex and ethnicity/race, the mortality rate is lowest among Pacific Islander/Asian women and highest among African American men [40, 41]. During the twentieth century, the total age-adjusted cancer mortality rate increased dramatically, reaching its peak at 215 cancer deaths per 100,000 people in 1991, primarily due to the smoking outbreak. By 2020, the prevalence had fallen to 152 per 100,000 due to smoking reductions, as well as advancements in early diagnosis and intervention. This declining trend resulted in more than 2.9 million cancer fatalities between 1991 and 2017, due to the gradual decline in mortality rate for the four major forms of cancer—prostate, breast, colorectal and lung. Cancer typically occurs in the elderly. Of all cancers in the USA, 80% of people aged 55 and over are diagnosed with cancer [42, 43]. Some habits also raise the risk, including smoking, alcohol consumption and excessive body weight. In the USA, about 39 in hundred women and 40 in hundred men get cancer in their lifetime [44–46].

Some features of cancer epidemiology and its natural course make it relatively easy to estimate mortality rates. The incidence of cancer is relatively constant over time. However, as the detection strategies differ over time, the incidence may suddenly increase due to enhanced detection. The prevalence of some cancer sites has increased in previous decades and has recently continued to decline significantly. One such instance of this is prostate cancer. The increase in the occurrence of brain cancer has also been the subject of speculation in the literature, though its growth has become less influenced by artefacts than that of prostate cancer. Sustainability, which indeed depends mainly on the development of new detection approaches and new therapies, changes very slowly [70–72, 75].

Variation in age-adjusted death rates is the main determinant of progress against cancer, though certain indicators, including the quality of life, are also essential. Since the early 1990s, the overall mortality rate due to cancer has decreased in the USA. According to the SEER Cancer Statistics Review report, death rates have also dropped significantly for several types of cancer. Although death rates from various forms of cancer have declined, the rates of some cancers have remained constant or even elevated. Conversely, the number of cancer survivors has increased due to the drop in overall cancer death rates. These findings suggest progress has been made against cancer, but further work needs to be done.

Declaration of Competing Interest The authors declare no conflicts of interest.

Acknowledgements The authors are grateful to the Ministry of Human Resource Development, Government of India for the financial support through *Scheme for Promotion of Academic and Research Collaboration* (*SPARC*) project "SPARC/2018-2019/P402/SL". We also acknowledge the support received from the National Research Foundation (NRF) of Korea for the Basic Science Research Program funded by the Ministry of Education (NRF-2019R1A6A1A03033215). We are grateful to SASTRA Deemed University, India and SKKU, South Korea for providing infrastructural support.

References

1. Izbicki T, Mazur J, Izbicka E (2003) Epidemiology and etiology of neuroblastoma: an overview. Anticancer Res 23:755–760
2. Bondy M, Ligon BL (1996) Epidemiology and etiology of intracranial meningiomas: a review. J Neuro-Oncol 29:197–205
3. Wirdefeldt K, Adami H-O, Cole P, Trichopoulos D, Mandel J (2011) Epidemiology and etiology of Parkinson's disease: a review of the evidence. Eur J Epidemiol 26:1
4. Rubin SC (2001) Cervical cancer: successes and failures. CA Cancer J Clin 51:89–91
5. Binnie WH (1976) A perspective of oral cancer: epidemiology and etiology of oral cancer in Britain. SAGE Publications, New York
6. Hui JYC (2016) Epidemiology and etiology of sarcomas. Surg Clin North Am 96:901–914
7. Wartenberg D, Groves FD, Adelman AS (2008) Acute lymphoblastic leukemia: epidemiology and etiology. In: Acute Leukemias. Springer, Berlin, pp 77–93
8. Ekström-Smedby K (2006) Epidemiology and etiology of non-Hodgkin lymphoma--a review. Acta Oncol (Madr) 45:258–271
9. Smedby KE, Hjalgrim H (2011) Epidemiology and etiology of mantle cell lymphoma and other non-Hodgkin lymphoma subtypes. Proc Seminars Cancer Biol 21:293–298
10. Bosch FX, Muñoz N (2002) The viral etiology of cervical cancer. Virus Res 89:183–190

11. Kessler II, Kulčar Ž, Zimolo A, Grgurević M, Strnad M, Goodwin BJ (1974) Cervical cancer in Yugoslavia. II. Epidemiologic factors of possible etiologic significance. J Natl Cancer Inst 53:51–60
12. Franco EL, Schlecht NF, Saslow D (2003) The epidemiology of cervical cancer. Cancer J 9:348–359
13. Reeves WC, Rawls WE, Brinton LA (1989) Epidemiology of genital papillomaviruses and cervical cancer. Rev Infect Dis 11:426–439
14. Brinton LA (1992) Epidemiology of cervical cancer--overview. IARC Sci Publ:3–23
15. Ansink AC, Heintz APM (1993) Epidemiology and etiology of squamous cell carcinoma of the vulva. Eur J Obstet Gynecol 48:111–115
16. Munoz N, Bosch X, Kaldor JM (1988) Does human papillomavirus cause cervical cancer? The state of the epidemiological evidence. Br J Cancer 57:1–5
17. Shanta V, Krishnamurthi S, Gajalakshmi CK, Swaminathan R, Ravichandran K (2000) Epidemiology of cancer of the cervix: global and national perspective. J Indian Med Assoc 98:49
18. Franco EL (1991) The sexually transmitted disease model for cervical cancer: incoherent epidemiologic findings and the role of misclassification of human papillomavirus infection. Epidemiology:98–106
19. Mohar A, Frias-Mendivil M (2000) Epidemiology of cervical cancer. Cancer Investig 18:584–590
20. Kessler II (1974) Cervical cancer epidemiology in historical perspective. J Reprod Med 12:173
21. Brinton LA, Fraumeni JF Jr (1986) Epidemiology of uterine cervical cancer. J Chronic Dis 39:1051–1065
22. Haverkos HW (2005) Multifactorial etiology of cervical cancer: a hypothesis. Medscape Gen Med 7:57
23. Schiffman M, Wentzensen N (2013) Human papillomavirus infection and the multistage carcinogenesis of cervical cancer. Cancer Epidemiol Prevention Biomarkers 22(4):553–560
24. Cohen SM, Shirai T, Steineck G (2000) Epidemiology and etiology of premalignant and malignant urothelial changes. Scand J Urol Nephrol 34:105–115
25. Bosch FX, de Sanjosé S (2007) The epidemiology of human papillomavirus infection and cervical cancer. Dis Markers 23:213–227
26. Johansson SL, Cohen SM (1997) Epidemiology and etiology of bladder cancer. Proc Seminars Surgical Oncol 13:291–298
27. Castellsagué X (2008) Natural history and epidemiology of HPV infection and cervical cancer. Gynecol Oncol 110:S4–S7
28. Bosch FX, Qiao Y-L, Castellsagué X (2006) Chapter 2 the epidemiology of human papillomavirus infection and its association with cervical cancer. Int J Gynecol Obstet 94:S8–S21
29. Gordis L, Gold EB (1993) Epidemiology and etiology of pancreatic cancer. Pancreas Biol. Pathobiol. Dis. Raven, New York, pp 837–855
30. Warwick GP, Harington JS (1973) Some aspects of the epidemiology and etiology of esophageal cancer with particular emphasis on the Transkei, South Africa. In: Advances in Cancer Research, vol 17. Elsevier, Amsterdam, pp 81–229
31. Ohgaki H, Kleihues P (2005) Epidemiology and etiology of gliomas. Acta Neuropathol 109:93–108
32. Deschler B, Lübbert M (2008) Acute myeloid leukemia: epidemiology and etiology. In: *Acute Leukemias*. Springer, Berlin, pp 47–56
33. Zunzunegui M-V, King M-C, Coria CF, Charlet J (1986) Male influences on cervical cancer risk. Am J Epidemiol 123:302–307
34. Naguib SM, Lundin FE, Davis HJ (1966) Relation of various epidemiologic factors to cervical cancer as determined by a screening program. Obstet Gynecol 28:451–459
35. Muggia FM (1990) Overview of cancer-related hypercalcemia: epidemiology and etiology. Proc Seminars Oncol 17:3–9
36. Wiemels J, Wrensch M, Claus EB (2010) Epidemiology and etiology of meningioma. J Neuro-Oncol 99:307–314

37. Cohen SM, Johansson SL (1992) Epidemiology and etiology of bladder cancer. Urol Clin North Am 19:421–428
38. Peterman TA, Jaffe HW, Beral V (1993) Epidemiologic clues to the etiology of Kaposi's sarcoma. AIDS 7:605–612
39. Franco EL (1991) Viral etiology of cervical cancer: a critique of the evidence. Rev Infect Dis 13:1195–1206
40. Heintz AP, Hacker NF, Lagasse LD (1985) Epidemiology and etiology of ovarian cancer: a review. Obstet Gynecol 66:127–135
41. Martin CE (1967) Epidemiology of cancer of the cervix. II. Marital and coital factors in cervical cancer. Am J Public Heal Nations Heal 57:803–814
42. Orem J, Mbidde EK, Lambert B, De Sanjose S, Weiderpass E (2007) Burkitt$\$'s lymphoma in Africa, a review of the epidemiology and etiology. Afr Health Sci 7
43. Busnardo B, De Vido D (2000) The epidemiology and etiology of differentiated thyroid carcinoma. Biomed Pharmacother 54:322–326
44. Beckett WS (1993) Epidemiology and etiology of lung cancer. Clin Chest Med 14:1
45. Gamliel Z (2000) Incidence, epidemiology, and etiology of esophageal cancer. Chest Surg Clin N Am 10:441–450
46. Tao Z, Shi A, Lu C, Song T, Zhang Z, Zhao J (2015) Breast cancer: epidemiology and etiology. Cell Biochem Biophys 72:333–338
47. Okuda K, Nakanuma Y, Miyazaki M (2002) Cholangiocarcinoma: recent progress. Part 1: epidemiology and etiology. J Gastroenterol Hepatol 17:1049–1055
48. Herrero R (1996) Epidemiology of cervical cancer. J Natl Cancer Inst Monogr 21:1–6
49. Bosch FX (2003) Epidemiology of human papillomavirus infections: new options for cervical cancer prevention. Salud Publica Mex 45:326–339
50. Trichopoulos D, Adami H-O, Ekbom A, Hsieh C-C, Lagiou P (2008) Early life events and conditions and breast cancer risk: from epidemiology to etiology. Int J Cancer 122:481–485
51. Maucort-Boulch D, Franceschi S, Plummer M (2008) International correlation between human papillomavirus prevalence and cervical cancer incidence. Cancer Epidemiol Prev Biomarkers 17:717–720
52. Denny L, Anorlu R (2012) Cervical cancer in Africa. Cancer Epidemiol Prev Biomarkers 21:1434–1438
53. Kesic V, Poljak M, Rogovskaya S (2012) Cervical cancer burden and prevention activities in Europe. Cancer Epidemiol Prev Biomarkers 21:1423–1433
54. Clarke MA, Wentzensen N, Mirabello L, Ghosh A, Wacholder S, Harari A, Lorincz A, Schiffman M, Burk RD (2012) Human papillomavirus DNA methylation as a potential biomarker for cervical cancer. Cancer Epidemiol Prev Biomarkers 21:2125–2137
55. Fang CY, Ma GX, Tan Y, Chi N (2007) A multifaceted intervention to increase cervical cancer screening among underserved Korean women. Cancer Epidemiol Prev Biomarkers 16:1298–1302
56. Yang N, Eijsink JJH, Lendvai Á, Volders HH, Klip H, Buikema HJ, van Hemel BM, Schuuring E, van der Zee AGJ, Wisman GBA (2009) Methylation markers for CCNA1 and C13ORF18 are strongly associated with high-grade cervical intraepithelial neoplasia and cervical cancer in cervical scrapings. Cancer Epidemiol Prev Biomarkers 18:3000–3007
57. Wentzensen N, von Knebel Doeberitz M (2007) Biomarkers in cervical cancer screening. Dis Markers 23:315–330
58. Arbyn M, Castle PE (2015) Offering self-sampling kits for HPV testing to reach women who do not attend in the regular cervical cancer screening program. Cancer Epidemiol Prev Biomarkers 24:769–772
59. Porras C, Rodríguez AC, Hildesheim A, Herrero R, González P, Wacholder S, Burk RD, Schiffman M (2009) Human papillomavirus types by age in cervical cancer precursors: predominance of human papillomavirus 16 in young women. Cancer Epidemiol Prev Biomarkers 18:863–865

60. Campbell CMP, Menezes LJ, Paskett ED, Giuliano AR (2012) Prevention of invasive cervical cancer in the United States: past, present, and future. Cancer Epidemiol Prev Biomarkers 21:1402–1408
61. Virtanen A, Nieminen P, Luostarinen T, Anttila A (2011) Self-sample HPV tests as an intervention for nonattendees of cervical cancer screening in Finland: a randomized trial. Cancer Epidemiol Prev Biomarkers 20:1960–1969
62. Hu X, Zhang Z, Ma D, Huettner PC, Massad LS, Nguyen L, Borecki I, Rader JS (2010) TP53, MDM2, NQO1, and susceptibility to cervical cancer. Cancer Epidemiol Prev Biomarkers 19:755–761
63. Coughlin SS, King J, Richards TB, Ekwueme DU (2006) Cervical cancer screening among women in metropolitan areas of the United States by individual-level and area-based measures of socioeconomic status, 2000 to 2002. Cancer Epidemiol Prev Biomarkers (15):2154–2159
64. Flatley JE, McNeir K, Balasubramani L, Tidy J, Stuart EL, Young TA, Powers HJ (2009) Folate status and aberrant DNA methylation are associated with HPV infection and cervical pathogenesis. Cancer Epidemiol Prev Biomarkers 18(10):2782–2789
65. Horner M-J, Altekruse SF, Zou Z, Wideroff L, Katki HA, Stinchcomb DG (2011) US geographic distribution of prevaccine era cervical cancer screening, incidence, stage, and mortality. Cancer Epidemiol Prev Biomarkers 20:591–599
66. Hemminki K, Chen B (2006) Familial risks for cervical tumors in full and half siblings: etiologic apportioning. Cancer Epidemiol Prev Biomarkers 15:1413–1414
67. Dasari S, Wudayagiri R, Valluru L (2015) Cervical cancer: biomarkers for diagnosis and treatment. Clin Chim Acta 445:7–11
68. Holmes RS, Hawes SE, Touré P, Dem A, Feng Q, Weiss NS, Kiviat NB (2009) HIV infection as a risk factor for cervical cancer and cervical intraepithelial neoplasia in Senegal. Cancer Epidemiol Prev Biomarkers 18:2442–2446
69. Murphy N, Ring M, Heffron C, King B, Killalea AG, Hughes C, Martin CM, McGuinness E, Sheils O, O'leary JJ (2005) p16INK4A, CDC6, and MCM5: predictive biomarkers in cervical preinvasive neoplasia and cervical cancer. J Clin Pathol 58:525–534
70. Waller J, Marlow LAV, Wardle J (2006) Mothers' attitudes towards preventing cervical cancer through human papillomavirus vaccination: a qualitative study. Cancer Epidemiol Prev Biomarkers 15:1257–1261
71. Tiro JA, Meissner HI, Kobrin S, Chollette V (2007) What do women in the US know about human papillomavirus and cervical cancer? Cancer Epidemiol Prev Biomarkers 16:288–294
72. Banerjee S, Karunagaran D (2019) An integrated approach for mining precise RNA-based cervical cancer staging biomarkers. Gene 712:143961
73. Wang JH, Sheppard VB, Schwartz MD, Liang W, Mandelblatt JS (2008) Disparities in cervical cancer screening between Asian American and non-Hispanic white women. Cancer Epidemiol Prev Biomarkers 17:1968–1973
74. Marlow LAV, Waller J, Wardle J (2009) The impact of human papillomavirus information on perceived risk of cervical cancer. Cancer Epidemiol Prev Biomarkers 18:373–376
75. Boulet GAV, Horvath CAJ, Berghmans S, Bogers J (2008) Human papillomavirus in cervical cancer screening: important role as biomarker. Cancer Epidemiol Prev Biomarkers 17:810–817

Cervical Cancer

2

Shrute Kannappan, Jung Heon Lee, Muthaiyan Lakshmanakumar, Noel Nesakumar, and John Bosco Balaguru Rayappan

Abstract

Cervical cancer ranks fourth among all types of cancers in women and accounts for close to 0.6 million new cases worldwide every year. Due to improvements in screening techniques, the mortality rate associated with cervical cancer has fallen

S. Kannappan
Department of Molecular Cell Biology, School of Medicine, Sungkyunkwan University (SKKU), Suwon, South Korea

Research Center for Advanced Materials Technology, Sungkyunkwan University (SKKU), Suwon, South Korea

J. H. Lee
School of Advanced Materials Science and Engineering, Research Center for Advanced Materials Technology, Biomedical Institute for Convergence at SKKU (BICS), Sungkyunkwan University (SKKU), Suwon, Republic of Korea

School of Advanced Materials Science and Engineering, Sungkyunkwan University (SKKU), Suwon, South Korea

Biomedical Institute for Convergence at SKKU (BICS), Sungkyunkwan University (SKKU), Suwon, South Korea

M. Lakshmanakumar · J. B. B. Rayappan (✉)
Centre for Nanotechnology and Advanced Biomaterials (CeNTAB), School of Electrical and Electronics Engineering, SASTRA Deemed University, Thanjavur, Tamil Nadu, India
e-mail: rjbosco@ece.sastra.edu

N. Nesakumar
Centre for Nanotechnology and Advanced Biomaterials (CeNTAB), SASTRA Deemed University, Thanjavur, Tamil Nadu, India

School of Chemical and Biotechnology, SASTRA Deemed University, Thanjavur, Tamil Nadu, India

J. B. B. Rayappan, J. H. Lee (eds.), *Biomarkers and Biosensors for Cervical Cancer Diagnosis*, https://doi.org/10.1007/978-981-16-2586-2_2

by around 50% worldwide. While cervical cancer is the leading cause of death among women in Africa, India and China attribute close to one-third of the total cases reported globally. Epidemiological studies suggest that the human papillomavirus (HPV) is the primary cause of cervical cancer. HPV is also responsible for anal, penile, vaginal, head, and neck cancers. HPV infection is very common that the risk of infection for women in the age of 15–80 years is 50–80%. Most of the HPV infections is cleared by the body inherently. In 10–20% of women, the virus persists and progresses into cervical intraepithelial neoplasm lesions by infecting the basal layer of keratinocytes. The infection metastasizes into an invasive cancer of the cervix upon expression of viral proteins E6, E7, which deregulate cell differentiation and proliferation. The HPV is the primary causative agent for cervical cancer and thus understanding the molecular biology and pathogenesis mechanism of the virus is discussed in this chapter.

Keywords

Genome · HPV · Pathogenesis · Molecular biology

2.1 Cervical Cancer

One of the most prevalent cancers among women is cervical cancer. According to the report of World Health Organization, 570,000 women with cervical cancer have been identified and approximately 311,000 women have died due to cervical cancer [1–4]. The American Cancer Society estimated that approximately 13,800 cases of invasive cervical cancer in 2020 and 4290 women were expected to die from cervical cancer in the USA. Invasive cervical cancer is found less commonly in the USA than cervical precancers. Cervical cancer has become one of the most leading causes of mortality among American women. Owing to the increased use of Pap tests, the mortality rate from cervical cancer has decreased considerably. The human papillomavirus (HPV) test has indeed been accepted as another standard test for the early diagnosis of cervical cancer in the past years, as nearly all cervical cancers are induced by HPV. The HPV test can be used alone or in conjunction with the Pap test as a co-test for identifying cervical cancer. Cervical cancer is commonly identified in women under the age of 44, with a mean age of 50 at the time of detection. Cervical cancer seldom grows in women under the age of 20 [3, 5, 6]. Many aged females do not recognize that there is still the possibility of developing cervical cancer as they get older. Nevertheless, cervical cancer rarely occurs in individuals who have had regular screening for cervical cancer before the age of 65. White, Native Alaskan, Native American, African American, and Hispanic women have been found to be particularly prone to cervical cancer in the USA.

A risk factor is something which increases the likelihood of a person getting cancer. While risk factors also affect cancer growth, most do not cause cancer explicitly. Only a few individuals with numerous risk factors rarely develop cancer, while the majority of people without risk factors develop cancer [1, 2, 7]. Exposure to diethylstilbestrol (DES), oral contraceptives, socioeconomic factors, age, smoking, herpes, immune system deficiency, and HPV infection are the main vital factors that can increase a woman's risk of getting cervical cancer. Among these, HPV infection is the most significant risk factor for cervical cancer. When most people are sexually active, there is a risk of getting infected with HPV. Conversely, most of the people eliminate the virus completely without any difficulty. There are more than 100 varieties of HPV. Most types of HPV are not linked to cancer, while only a few types of HPV are linked to cancer [8–10]. At least 14 types of HPV have been found to cause cervical cancer, which is regarded as high risk. HPV18 and HPV16 are the most common strains or types of HPV linked with cervical cancer. HPV16 and HPV18 are responsible for causing more than 70% of precancerous cervical lesions and cervical cancers. There is also scientific proof that HPV is directly connected to cancers of oropharynx, penis, vagina, vulva, and anus. Having numerous sex partners or trying to have intercourse at a younger age puts a person at a greater risk of getting infected with high-risk types of HPV. Conversely, individuals with lower immune systems are at increased risk of experiencing cervical cancer. Human immunodeficiency virus (HIV), a virus that tends to cause acquired immunodeficiency syndrome, treatments for other types of cancer, organ transplantation, and corticosteroids can induce a weakened immune system [11–13]. Specifically, when a female possesses HIV, her immune system is less capable of fighting premature cancer. Moreover, people with genetic herpes are known to have an increased risk of cervical cancer. When it comes to smoking, females who regularly smoke are significantly more likely to experience cervical cancer than females who do not smoke. In contrast, there are rare cases of cervical cancer in people under the age of 20. The risk of developing cervical cancer increases in late adolescents and those under 30 [14–16]. Females in this age category remain vulnerable and undertake periodic screenings for cervical cancer, including an HPV test and/or a Pap test. Young women who have had cervical cancer are the least likely to be directly exposed to screening for cervical cancer. Women from low-income households, Native American women, Hispanic women, and black women are the people most vulnerable to cervical cancer. A few research findings indicate that an increased risk of cervical cancer may be linked to birth control pills. Nevertheless, perhaps extensive investigation is required to recognize how birth control pill use is directly linked to the progression of cervical cancer [17–20]. Females whose mothers were provided this medication during pregnancy to avoid premature birth have had a greater risk of having a specific type of cervical or vaginal cancer when exposed to DES is involved. DES was offered from around 1940 until 1970 for this particular reason. Females subjected to DES must have an annual screening test that contains a 4-quadrant Pap test and also a cervical Pap test, wherein specimens of cells from across all corners of the vagina are collected to inspect for abnormal cells [21–23].

There are organizations in developed countries that allow women to get the HPV vaccine and women to get tested regularly. Testing enables the identification of precancerous lesions at different phases as they can be easily treated. Early diagnosis in each of these countries can prevent up to 80% of cervical cancers [24–26]. Restricted access to these prevention strategies is available in developing countries, but cervical cancer sometimes goes unrecognized until it has progressed and symptoms appear. Additionally, in developing countries, access to healthcare for women with cervical cancer is constrained, leading to increased mortality rates due to cervical cancer [27–29].

2.2 Pathology

2.2.1 Molecular Biology: HPV Genome Organization

The human papillomavirus, which belongs to the family of *Papovaviridae,* is a non-enveloped, icosahedral DNA based virus consisting of one copy of double-stranded DNA of about 7900 bases [30]. HPV is a rather small virus with an average diameter of 60 nm, bearing a resemblance to a golf ball when viewed under an electron microscope [31]. While the virus is double-stranded, only one of the strands (coding strand) is used as a template for transcription, which can be functionally classified into the non-coding region (LCR, long coding region), early region (E1-E8, except E4), and the late region (E4, capsid proteins) [32]. The HPV genome consists of a total of 10 ORFs (open reading frames), constitutively forming the early and late regions [33] (Fig. 2.1).

The E1 region codes for the only enzyme transcribed by the HPV—ATP-dependent DNA helicase which plays a vital role in the replication of the virus [35]. The E2 gene is a key player in regulating viral transcription and replication, being one of the most conserved HPV domains [36]. A unique feature of the E2 region is its ability to act as either an activator or a repressor depending on which site it binds to. While the full-length E2 (E2TA) is a trans-activator that binds to the E2 activation domain, the truncated E2 competes with E2TA for the DNA binding site and renders E2TA inactive [37]. The truncated E2 binds close to the E6/E7 promoter region, resulting in the repression of transcription [38]. Conversely, the E4 ORF is found within the E2 ORF, is reported to play a vital role in the HPV genome amplification by forming a fusion protein with E1 (E1^E4) [39]. Despite weak transforming activity showcased by the HPV E5 transmembrane protein, they promote carcinogenesis due to their high mitogenic activity, the ability to evade the immune system, and inhibit apoptosis [40].

The E6/E7 ORFs are solely responsible for the oncogenic properties of HPV. Particularly, the high risk HPV E6 ORF does so by activating telomerase, p53 (tumor suppressor) inhibition by acetylation and transactivation, pRb inactivation causing immortalization of cells, immune evasion resulting in protection from apoptosis [41]. On similar lines, the hr-HPV E7 protein is also oncogenic in the sense that its primary role is to interact with tumor suppressors (pRb, retinoblastoma), resulting in escape from cell cycle arrest [30]. The late region is the most conserved sequence among HPV genotypes that code for the major capsid protein L1 and the minor capsid protein L2, which combine to form 72 capsomers [42].

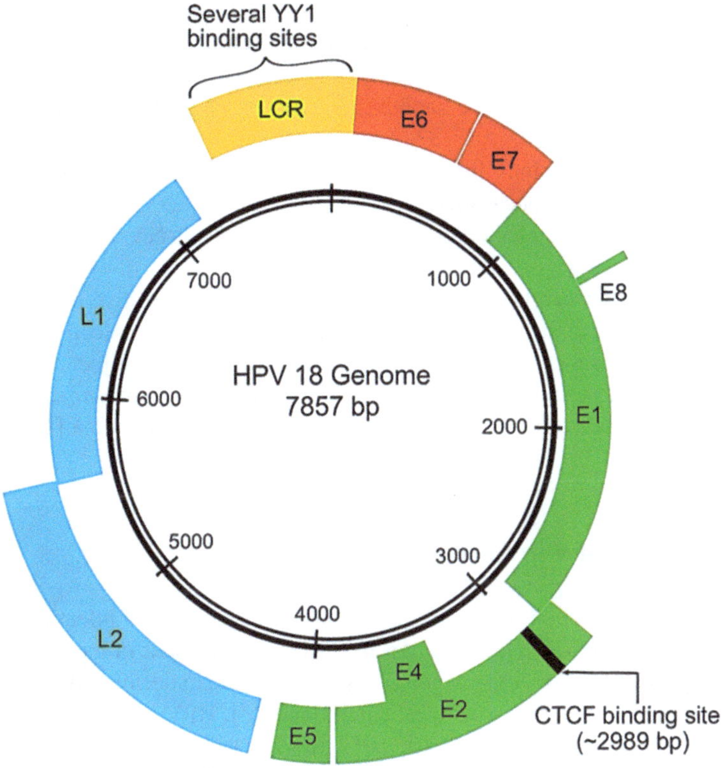

Fig. 2.1 HPV genome organization [34] (Copyright Received)

2.2.2 Life Cycle of HPV: Virus Replication—Latent to Productive Infection

Broadly, the HPV multiplication cycle can be categorized into latent infection and productive infection. The following is a brief overview of the conspicuous events involved in HPV multiplication:

(1) HPV enters the basal stem cells (only cells in the squamous epithelium that can divide) of the epithelium via an intraepithelial lesion [31].
(2) HPV enters into the basal cells through heparan sulfate proteoglycans (HSPGs) with the expression of L1 (initial attachment) and further L2 is expressed as the virion binds to the cell surface [32].
(3) Endocytosis and release of the viral DNA into the nucleus guided by L2 (NLS, nuclear localization signal) [43].
(4) Genome amplification with the help of E1, E2 aids fast replication of all viral genes and maintenance as low copy number episomes [44].
(5) With the increase in viral copy number in undifferentiated cells (switch to rolling circle replication), daughter cells migrate to the suprabasal cells with expression

E6, E7 oncogenes, resulting in the inhibition of proliferation of basal cells while favoring hyperproliferation of the healthy suprabasal cells, resulting in accumulation of genomic mutations [45].
(6) Expression of E1, E2 in the suprabasal layer causing a further increase in the viral copy number.
(7) Cell cycle exit, terminal differentiation of HPV with the expression of L1, L2 aiding nucleocapsid encapsulation of viral DNA [46].
(8) Virion release from infected squamous epithelial cells is aided by E4 ORF [39].

The fine line between latent multiplication cycles and vegetative infection cycle happens in the fourth step [44]. While in the case of a latent infection, the virus replicates in the basal cells solely for its maintenance, with the influence of various exogenous and endogenous factors, it may evolve into a vegetative infection affecting the differentiated cells, eventually resulting in invasive carcinoma [47].

2.2.3 Role of HPV in Cervical Cancer

From the previous section, it can thus be ascertained that an HPV infection does not imply the presence of CC. However, it is the differentiation state of the host cells and the strain of the infecting virus, which plays a primal role in deciding the probability of it developing into invasive cervical carcinoma [48]. HPV can be categorized as high-risk HPV (hr-HPV) or low-risk HPV (lr-HPV) depending on the probable outcome of the infection. While HPV-16, 18, 31, 33, 35, 39, 45, 51, 52, 56, 58, 59, 68, and 73, 82 account for the hr-HPV types which possess oncogenic potential, the lr-HPV subtypes 6, 11, 42, 43, and 44 are responsible for the formation of anogenital condylomas but, in exceptional cases, may also progress to invasive carcinoma [49].

Based on the multiplication cycle of HPV, it is evident that the virus migrates from the basal cells (bottom) towards the surface. Thus, based on histology, a productive HPV infection can be classified into various stages as follows:

1. Cervical lesions/squamous intraepithelial lesions (SIL) based on the Bethesda classification are further classified as:
   (i) LSIL (low-grade SIL) which is a mild dysplasia causing a condyloma or cervical intraepithelial neoplasia (CIN-1) characteristic of high viral replication rate with mild cellular alterations.
   (ii) HSIL (high-grade SIL) where the viral replication rate is lower with increased cancerous cell proliferation and lower cellular maturation (CIN-2, CIN-3).

The qualifying characteristic for a CIN is the presence of a nuclear abnormality. Each of the CIN types affects a third of the epithelium, i.e. CIN-1 affects one-third of the bottom-most part of the epithelium, while CIN-3 affects one-third of the top.

2. Carcinoma in situ is the stage where CIN3 covers the entire width of the epithelium.
3. Invasive carcinoma or the final stage, is where infiltration into the uterine muscles takes place, further metastasizing throughout the body [48].

Mostly, only a latent infection (only the expression of the E1 and E2 genes) prevails and is thus generally removed from the body by a good immune system [50]. In 90% of cases within 12–18 months of infection, the infection is cleared via cell-mediated adaptive immune response and weak humoral response evoked by L1 [51]. However, when the viral genes integrate into the host genome, the integration happens at sites of proto-oncogenes such as C-Myc (tumor suppressor), playing a role in carcinogenesis [52]. Since HPV is a circular virus, it requires linearization for integration into the host genome. It has been reported that the cut happens in the E1, E2 ORF [53]. But since E2 helps in the inhibition of the E6 and E7 oncoproteins, this results in the overexpression of oncoproteins, leading to the inactivation of tumor suppression proteins.

As mentioned earlier, E6 targets p53, while E7 targets pRb resulting in the escape of cells from cell cycle arrest, eventually leading to the build-up of genetic mutations [54]. As a consequence of these events, the activation of transcription factor E2-F, cyclins, CDKs (cyclin-dependent kinases) acts as activators for DNA replication further promoting proliferation [55]. Besides, the HPV multiplication cycle has evolved in such a way that the replication processes happen deep inside the epithelial layers that eliminates an immune attack trigger from the picture. Only when the virions are released at later stages of the infection, they do encounter the immune system, but they again evade the immune system through various mechanisms. This includes the downregulation of CDH-1 by E6 causing an inability for the host immune cells to allow viral antigen presentation, inhibition of TLR-9 by E5 resulting in lower APC (antigen-presenting cells) attraction, and downregulation of TAP-1 by E7 causing lower T_c cell activation, to name a few.

2.3 Conclusion

It is thus evident that HPV is the primary causative agent for CC and thus, understanding the molecular biology and pathogenesis of the virus is paramount in terms of prognosis, diagnosis, and choosing appropriate therapeutic interventions to combat the infection. It is also important to note that the presence of an HPV infection does not guarantee the presence of CC, but rather the stage of infection, which ascertains CC. In spite of years of work, important aspects of CC progression and transformation are yet to be unveiled given the complexity of HPV infection. Thus, scope for future studies in understanding the pathogenesis will pave the way for a vaccine to completely eradicate CC.

Declaration of Competing Interest The authors declare no conflicts of interest.

Acknowledgements The authors are grateful to the Ministry of Human Resource Development, Government of India for the financial support through *Scheme for Promotion of Academic and Research Collaboration* (*SPARC*) project "SPARC/2018-2019/P402/SL." We also acknowledge the support received from the National Research Foundation (NRF) of Korea for the Basic Science Research Program funded by the Ministry of Education (NRF-2019R1A6A1A03033215). We are grateful to SASTRA Deemed University, India and SKKU, South Korea for providing infrastructural support.

References

1. Wang JH, Sheppard VB, Schwartz MD, Liang W, Mandelblatt JS (2008) Disparities in cervical cancer screening between Asian American and non-Hispanic white women. Cancer Epidemiol Prev Biomarkers 17:1968–1973
2. Murphy N, Ring M, Heffron C, King B, Killalea AG, Hughes C, Martin CM, McGuinness E, Sheils O, O'leary JJ (2005) p16INK4A, CDC6, and MCM5: predictive biomarkers in cervical preinvasive neoplasia and cervical cancer. J Clin Pathol 58:525–534
3. Holmes RS, Hawes SE, Touré P, Dem A, Feng Q, Weiss NS, Kiviat NB (2009) HIV infection as a risk factor for cervical cancer and cervical intraepithelial neoplasia in Senegal. Cancer Epidemiol Prev Biomarkers 18:2442–2446
4. Dasari S, Wudayagiri R, Valluru L (2015) Cervical cancer: biomarkers for diagnosis and treatment. Clin Chim Acta 445:7–11
5. Horner M-J, Altekruse SF, Zou Z, Wideroff L, Katki HA, Stinchcomb DG (2011) US geographic distribution of prevaccine era cervical cancer screening, incidence, stage, and mortality. Cancer Epidemiol Prev Biomarkers 20:591–599
6. Hemminki K, Chen B (2006) Familial risks for cervical tumors in full and half siblings: etiologic apportioning. Cancer Epidemiol Prev Biomarkers 15:1413–1414
7. Marlow LAV, Waller J, Wardle J (2009) The impact of human papillomavirus information on perceived risk of cervical cancer. Cancer Epidemiol Prev Biomarkers 18:373–376
8. Banerjee S, Karunagaran D (2019) An integrated approach for mining precise RNA-based cervical cancer staging biomarkers. Gene 712:143961
9. Boulet GAV, Horvath CAJ, Berghmans S, Bogers J (2008) Human papillomavirus in cervical cancer screening: important role as biomarker. Cancer Epidemiol Prev Biomarkers 17:810–817
10. Tornesello ML, Buonaguro L, Giorgi-Rossi P, Buonaguro FM (2013) Viral and cellular biomarkers in the diagnosis of cervical intraepithelial neoplasia and cancer. Biomed Res Int 2013
11. Ohgaki H, Kleihues P (2005) Epidemiology and etiology of gliomas. Acta Neuropathol 109:93–108
12. Warwick GP, Harington JS (1973) Some aspects of the epidemiology and etiology of esophageal cancer with particular emphasis on the Transkei, South Africa. In: Advances in cancer research, vol 17. Elsevier, Amsterdam, pp 81–229
13. Gordis L, Gold EB (1993) Epidemiology and etiology of pancreatic cancer. Pancreas Biol. Pathobiol. Dis. Raven, New York, pp 837–855
14. Castellsagué X (2008) Natural history and epidemiology of HPV infection and cervical cancer. Gynecol Oncol 110:S4–S7
15. Bosch FX, Qiao Y-L, Castellsagué X (2006) CHAPTER 2 the epidemiology of human papillomavirus infection and its association with cervical cancer. Int J Gynecol Obstet 94:S8–S21
16. Johansson SL, Cohen SM (1997) Epidemiology and etiology of bladder cancer. Proc Seminars Surg Oncol 13:291–298

17. Bosch FX, de Sanjosé S (2007) The epidemiology of human papillomavirus infection and cervical cancer. Dis Markers 23:213–227
18. Cohen SM, Shirai T, Steineck G (2000) Epidemiology and etiology of premalignant and malignant urothelial changes. Scand J Urol Nephrol 34:105–115
19. Haverkos HW (2005) Multifactorial etiology of cervical cancer: a hypothesis. Medscape Gen Med 7:57
20. Schiffman M, Wentzensen N (2013) Human papillomavirus infection and the multistage carcinogenesis of cervical cancer. Cancer Epidemiol Prev Biomarkers 22(4):553–560
21. Franco EL (1991) The sexually transmitted disease model for cervical cancer: incoherent epidemiologic findings and the role of misclassification of human papillomavirus infection. Epidemiology 2:98–106
22. Shanta V, Krishnamurthi S, Gajalakshmi CK, Swaminathan R, Ravichandran K (2000) Epidemiology of cancer of the cervix: global and national perspective. J Indian Med Assoc 98:49
23. Munoz N, Bosch X, Kaldor JM (1988) Does human papillomavirus cause cervical cancer? The state of the epidemiological evidence. Br J Cancer 57:1–5
24. Ansink AC, Heintz APM (1993) Epidemiology and etiology of squamous cell carcinoma of the vulva. Eur J Obstet Gynecol 48:111–115
25. Reeves WC, Rawls WE, Brinton LA (1989) Epidemiology of genital papillomaviruses and cervical cancer. Rev Infect Dis 11:426–439
26. Brinton LA (1992) Epidemiology of cervical cancer--overview. IARC Sci Publ:3–23
27. Binnie WH (1976) A perspective of oral cancer: epidemiology and etiology of oral cancer in Britain. SAGE Publications, Thousand Oaks
28. Rubin SC (2001) Cervical cancer: successes and failures. CA Cancer J Clin 51:89–91
29. Wirdefeldt K, Adami H-O, Cole P, Trichopoulos D, Mandel J (2011) Epidemiology and etiology of Parkinson's disease: a review of the evidence. Eur J Epidemiol 26:1
30. Roman A, Munger K (2013) The papillomavirus E7 proteins. Virology 445:138–168. https://doi.org/10.1016/j.virol.2013.04.013
31. Egawa K (2003) Do human papillomaviruses target epidermal stem cells? Dermatology 207:251–254. https://doi.org/10.1159/000073085
32. Schäfer G, Blumenthal MJ, Katz AA (2015) Interaction of human tumor viruses with host cell surface receptors and cell entry. Viruses 7:2592–2617. https://doi.org/10.3390/v7052592
33. Knipe DM, Howley P (2013) Fields virology, 6th edn. Wolters Kluwer/Lippincott Williams & Wilkins Health, Philadelphia, PA; ISBN 9781451105636
34. Kroupis C, Vourlidis N (2011) Human papilloma virus (HPV) molecular diagnostics. Clin Chem Lab Med 49:1783–1799. https://doi.org/10.1515/CCLM.2011.685
35. Bergvall M, Melendy T, Archambault J (2013) The E1 proteins. Virology 445:35–56. https://doi.org/10.1016/j.virol.2013.07.020
36. Mcbride AA (2013) The papillomavirus E2 proteins. Virology 445:57–79. https://doi.org/10.1016/j.virol.2013.06.006
37. Lim DA, Gossen M, Lehman CW, Botchan MR (1998) Competition for DNA binding sites between the short and long forms of E2 dimers underlies repression in bovine papillomavirus type 1 DNA replication control. J Virol 72:1931–1940
38. Bernard BA, Bailly C, Lenoir MC, Darmon M, Thierry F, Yaniv M (1989) The human papillomavirus type 18 (HPV18) E2 gene product is a repressor of the HPV18 regulatory region in human keratinocytes. J Virol 63:4317 LP–4314324
39. Doorbar J (2013) The E4 protein; structure, function and patterns of expression. Virology 445:80–98. https://doi.org/10.1016/j.virol.2013.07.008
40. DiMaio D, Petti LM (2013) The E5 proteins. Virology 445:99–114. https://doi.org/10.1016/j.virol.2013.05.006
41. Vande Pol SB, Klingelhutz AJ (2013) Papillomavirus E6 oncoproteins. Virology 445:115–137. https://doi.org/10.1016/j.virol.2013.04.026
42. Klug A, Finch JT (1965) Structure of viruses of the papilloma-polyoma type: I. human wart virus. J Mol Biol 11:403–IN44. https://doi.org/10.1016/S0022-2836(65)80066-3

43. Broniarczyk J, Massimi P, Bergant M, Banks L (2015) Human papillomavirus infectious entry and trafficking is a rapid process. J Virol 89:8727–8732. https://doi.org/10.1128/JVI.00722-15
44. Maglennon GA, McIntosh P, Doorbar J (2011) Persistence of viral DNA in the epithelial basal layer suggests a model for papillomavirus latency following immune regression. Virology 414:153–163. https://doi.org/10.1016/j.virol.2011.03.019
45. Doorbar J, Quint W, Banks L, Bravo IG, Stoler M, Broker TR, Stanley MA (2012) The biology and life-cycle of human papillomaviruses. Vaccine 30:F55–F70. https://doi.org/10.1016/j.vaccine.2012.06.083
46. Conway MJ, Meyers C (2009) Replication and assembly of human papillomaviruses. J Dent Res 88:307–317. https://doi.org/10.1177/0022034509333446
47. Fehrmann F, Laimins LA (2003) Human papillomaviruses: targeting differentiating epithelial cells for malignant transformation. Oncogene 22:5201–5207. https://doi.org/10.1038/sj.onc.1206554
48. Tadlaoui KA, Hassou N, Bennani B, Ennaji MM (2019) Emergence of oncogenic high-risk human papillomavirus types and cervical cancer. Elsevier Inc., Amsterdam; ISBN 9780128194003
49. Muñoz N, Bosch FX, De Sanjosé S, Herrero R, Castellsagué X, Shah KV, Snijders PJF, Meijer CJLM (2003) Epidemiologic classification of human papillomavirus types associated with cervical cancer. N Engl J Med 348:518–527. https://doi.org/10.1056/NEJMoa021641
50. Infections génitales à HPV (2006) Bases fondamentales. In: Infections à papillomavirus: État des connaissances, pratiques et prévention vaccinale. Springer, Paris, pp 3–45. ISBN 978-2-287-33480-1
51. Plummer M, Schiffman M, Castle PE, Maucort-Boulch D, Wheeler CM (2007) A 2-year prospective study of human papillomavirus persistence among women with a cytological diagnosis of atypical squamous cells of undetermined significance or low-grade squamous intraepithelial lesion. J Infect Dis 195:1582–1589. https://doi.org/10.1086/516784
52. Peter M, Rosty C, Couturier J, Radvanyi F, Teshima H, Sastre-Garau X (2006) MYC activation associated with the integration of HPV DNA at the MYC locus in genital tumors. Oncogene 25:5985–5993. https://doi.org/10.1038/sj.onc.1209625
53. Arias-Pulido H, Peyton CL, Joste NE, Vargas H, Wheeler CM (2006) Human papillomavirus type 16 integration in cervical carcinoma in situ and in invasive cervical cancer. J Clin Microbiol 44:1755–1762. https://doi.org/10.1128/JCM.44.5.1755-1762.2006
54. Münger K, Howley PM (2002) Human papillomavirus immortalization and transformation functions. Virus Res 89:213–228. https://doi.org/10.1016/s0168-1702(02)00190-9
55. Burd EM (2003) Human papillomavirus and cervical cancer. Clin Microbiol Rev 16:1–17. https://doi.org/10.1128/CMR.16.1.1

Potential Biomarkers for Early Diagnosis of Cervical Cancer

3

Shrute Kannappan, Jung Heon Lee, Muthaiyan Lakshmanakumar, John Bosco Balaguru Rayappan, and Noel Nesakumar

Abstract

Biomarkers provide a platform to aid early detection, diagnosis, prognosis, and prediction of the disease. In the case of cervical cancer, the biomarkers primarily serve to identify the viral infection at a precancerous stage in order to aid in early

S. Kannappan
Department of Molecular Cell Biology, School of Medicine, Sungkyunkwan University (SKKU), Suwon, South Korea

Research Center for Advanced Materials Technology, Sungkyunkwan University (SKKU), Suwon, South Korea

J. H. Lee
School of Advanced Materials Science and Engineering, Research Center for Advanced Materials Technology, Biomedical Institute for Convergence at SKKU (BICS), Sungkyunkwan University (SKKU), Suwon, Republic of Korea

School of Advanced Materials Science and Engineering, Sungkyunkwan University (SKKU), Suwon, South Korea

Biomedical Institute for Convergence at SKKU (BICS), Sungkyunkwan University (SKKU), Suwon, South Korea

M. Lakshmanakumar · J. B. B. Rayappan
Centre for Nanotechnology and Advanced Biomaterials (CeNTAB), School of Electrical and Electronics Engineering, SASTRA Deemed University, Thanjavur, Tamil Nadu, India

N. Nesakumar (✉)
Centre for Nanotechnology and Advanced Biomaterials (CeNTAB), SASTRA Deemed University, Thanjavur, Tamil Nadu, India

School of Chemical and Biotechnology, SASTRA Deemed University, Thanjavur, Tamil Nadu, India
e-mail: noel@scbt.sastra.edu

J. B. B. Rayappan, J. H. Lee (eds.), *Biomarkers and Biosensors for Cervical Cancer Diagnosis*, https://doi.org/10.1007/978-981-16-2586-2_3

intervention. They are broadly classified into molecular markers (nucleic acid based) and protein-based markers. Nucleic acid-based molecular markers are primarily based on the detection of HPV as the integration of HPV DNA into the host genome is a critical player in progression of the tumor. In addition, specific DNA loci in the human genome are also reported to have global and local epigenetic variation in the presence of HPV infection and thus act as suitable biomarkers. Less common but reliable nucleic acid-based markers include analysis of non-coding RNA such as miRNA, circular RNA (circRNA), and long non-coding RNA (lncRNA). The non-coding RNA and epigenetics-based screening platforms are currently at a nascent stage and thence further basic science research is essential to prove their clinical applicability. Protein-based biomarkers include differentially expressed host protein due to the influence of HPV oncoproteins. These biomarkers broadly fall into the categories of cell cycle regulators (KIF11, DTL), tumor suppressors (CBX7, KLK10), or proto-oncogenes (HBXIP, SMC4). Thence, an in-depth evaluation of the molecular and protein-based biomarkers will pave the way to affordable, simple, selective, and specific detection of cervical cancer at an early stage.

Keywords

HPV biomarkers · Cervical cancer biomarkers · circRNA HPV · miRNA HPV · lncRNA HPV

3.1 Introduction

Cervical cancer is a major burden in the healthcare industry, accounting for close to 0.6 million new cases every year worldwide, ranking fourth among cancers caused in women [1]. A critical key to tackling the disease at a global level is the implementation of large-scale screening techniques, adopting effective strategies to specifically identify the viral infection (Human papillomavirus—HPV) at an early stage. Over the years, various research groups have extensively worked on identifying specific biosignatures in response to an HPV infection and thus correlating them with the various stages of cervical cancer (CC). According to the National Institute of Health, these biosignatures/biomarkers are defined as "*A biological molecule found in blood, other body fluids, or tissues that is a sign of a normal or abnormal process, or of a condition or disease*" [2]. These biomarkers are tools that provide a platform to aid early detection, diagnosis, prognosis, and prediction of the outcome of the patients.

As described in the previous chapter, the presence of an HPV infection does not imply the development into invasive cancer. In more than 90% of cases with an HPV infection, the virus is generally cleared from the body within about 2–3 years [3]. Only in a small percentage of the population (less than 8%) with a rather compromised immune system (inclusive of but not restricted to), the infections transform into cervical lesions which further develop into carcinoma in situ and then metastasize into a fully blown carcinoma of the cervix [4]. Thus, an ideal biomarker should be able to accurately unmask the infection at a precancerous lesion stage given the higher probability for it to transform into an invasive carcinoma thus providing a chance for intervention early on, improving the disease management. Identification of stage-dependent biomarkers (risk assessment) that can distinguish between transient and clinically significant infections can thus be cited as a critical necessity for the detection of cervical cancer, particularly. This is further substantiated by the fact that the treatment course depends on the grade of the infection. In addition to the use of biomarkers for screening the early onset of disease, it is used in every stage of the disease, surveillance of treatment response and possible prognosis to ascertain the outcomes of the patients on a case by case basis.

The biomarkers for cervical cancer are broadly classified into molecular markers and protein-based markers. The molecular markers can further be subdivided into DNA and RNA based markers which are characteristic of either the virus or the host.

3.2 Molecular Markers

3.2.1 DNA Based Markers

Since the publication of the DNA sequence of the HPV in the late 1980s, one of the initial biomarkers for the detection of CC was the identification of HPV DNA in various samples [5]. Radiolabeled DNA probes were used in cervical smears or scrapes using a dot-blot assay. Shortly following this was the in situ hybridization using non-radiolabeled fluorescent probes.

One such early study reports in situ hybridization for the detection of the HPV type 1a, 6b, 16, 11 using synthetically designed 30-mers labeled with biotin targeting the beginning of the E6 open reading frame. The study was able to successfully differentiate type specificity between the HPV-16 and HPV-11 strains whose probes differed only by four bases with minimal cross-hybridization. The total detection time of 2 h (which was essentially just comprised of the incubation time) paved a way towards an easy, safe (in comparison with radiolabeled detection techniques), and an efficient HPV detection system [6]. In addition to the in situ hybridization detection of HPV in cervical smears, attempts to closely follow this have also been made to identify HPV in Cervical Intraepithelial Neoplasia (CIN) as well [7].

Initially, the identification of HPV DNA in cervical tissue samples was due to the idea that the integration of the HPV genome into the host precedes the development of lesions into invasive carcinoma. However, with years of research, it is now widely accepted that the progression into CC precedes the integration process. Thus, alternative biomarkers are being studied to effectively diagnose CC [8].

Epigenetics is defined as the study of variations happening in a heritable phenotype without changes in the DNA sequence [9]. Methylation and acetylation of DNA are the most common chemical modifications which result in altered gene expression. The methylation sites are predominantly Cytosine, Guanine based which may or may not be a part of the CpG islands [10]. In a typical cancer of cancer cells—

hypomethylation is observed genome-wide while hypermethylation is observed at the promoter regions resulting in inactivation of tumor-suppressive genes [11].

The expression levels of the HPV L1 protein play a major role in determining the grade of a CIN and the probability of it progressing to CC. As the L1 protein, which codes for the nucleocapsid, is strongly immunogenic—the basal cells downregulate the L1 protein primarily in the case of a productive infection while not in the case of a low-grade lesion [12]. Thus, since gene regulation plays a major role in the progression of the infection, primarily epigenetic modifications such as methylation of the L1 genes come into the picture as they are characteristic of the integration of viral genes into the host genome [13]. The analysis of L1 genes rather than the conventional analysis of LCR (late coding regions) has also been shown to be more powerful since the latter is largely influenced by the physical state of the virus [14].

A pyrosequencing-based study of exfoliated cervical cells collected from a Thai female population suggests the scope of using the methylation status of the HPV 16 L1 gene (with specific emphasis on the 5′ and 3′ ends of the gene) as a marker to understand infection progression, as is evident from the following figure (Fig. 3.1a). A clear distinction between CIN1 and the following stages can be made by analyzing the hypermethylation status of the 5′CpG islands 5609 and 5600, while only a comparatively lower methylation % can be found in the 3′ terminus CpG islands of the L1 gene. Thus, the combined analysis of %methylation of the sites 5600 and 5609 from exfoliated cervical cells can be used as a prognostic marker for CC, chiefly to differentiate CIN2–3 from CC [15].

In addition to the analysis of HPV specific genes methylation status, the global DNA methylation profile of various tumor suppressor genes also provides an overall picture of the status of lesions. Based on quantitative methylation-specific PCR, it was concluded that, out of the 15 genes taken into consideration for analysis, hypermethylation of hsa-miR-124, SOX1, TERT, and LMX1A was deemed to be the independent predictors (95% confidence interval) of CIN2+ regardless of HPV status (Fig. 3.1b) [16].

Quantitative-methylation specific PCR, which offers sensitivity equal to the HPV DNA test, reveals that hsa-miR-124 helps improve cell adhesion due to its role in inducing expression of insulin-growth factor, while LMX1A has a role in aiding epithelial–mesenchymal transition (EMT), which is an important trademark of cancer. The study has also hypothesized an alternative method in the overall cervical carcinogenesis pathway, suggesting that even after the clearance of HPV from the system, the initial hypermethylation caused by the virus could have an impact on its progress to a high-grade lesion [16]. Thus, providing substantial evidence that unlike the traditional study of epigenetic changes in the genome, studies on miRNA could help to identify novel biomarkers of CC. A few other epigenetic based markers for CC are described in Table 3.1.

The epigenetic based biomarkers are still far from being used in commercial assays, primarily since the assays utilized for identifying these methylation patterns are not well standardized, resulting in the detection of false-positive markers and

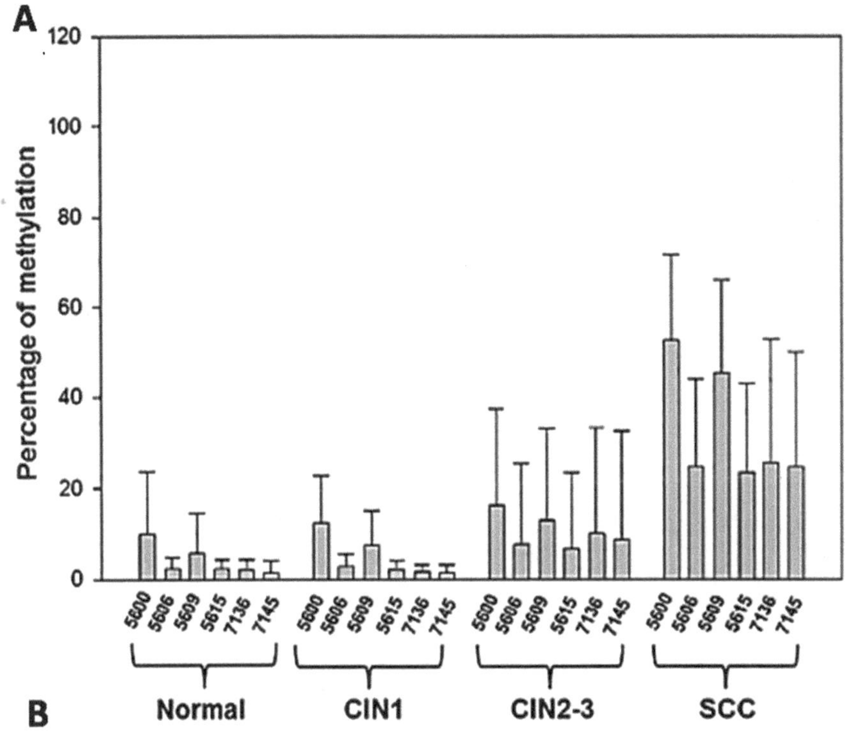

B

Variable	Category	N	OR (*)	95% CI (OR)
Hr-HPV	Negative	149	1.0	Reference
	Positive	253	5.5	(2.6–11.6)
hsa-miR-124-2	Unmethylated	185	1.0	Reference
	Methylated (>4.5)	217	5.1	(2.5–10.3)
SOX1	Unmethylated	271	1.0	Reference
	Methylated (>14.4)	131	2.8	(1.4–5.3)
TERT	Unmethylated	261	1.0	Reference
	Methylated (>1.2)	141	2.2	(1.2–4.1)
LMX1A	Unmethylated	319	1.0	Reference
	Methylated (>2.5)	83	2.0	(1.03–3.9)

OR: odds ratio; 95% CI: 95% confidence interval. Note: the cutoff of PMR values were defined by ROC curve analysis. (*) Model adjusted by age (continuous variable).

Fig. 3.1 (**a**) Stage dependent methylation status variation of HPV 16 L1 gene [15]. (**b**) Proposed independent predictors of CIN2+ based on global methylation patterns [16]. (Copyrights Received)

large variability. Besides, unlike the limited number of RNA based markers, the number of sites where DNA methylation can take place is extremely diverse, so it further complicates analysis [24].

Table 3.1 List of methylation pattern-based biomarkers for cervical cancer detection

S. No.	Biomarker	Organism	Function of biomarker	Clinical implication	Regulation pattern	Clinical samples	Reference
1	SOX1, TERT, LMX1A	Host	Tumor suppressing activity	Independent indicator for detection of precancer lesions/CIN2+ (irrespective of HPV status)/high-grade SIL	Hyper	447	[16]
2	GHSR, ASCL, LHX8, SST, ZIC1	Host	Methylation markers—No specific function		Hyper	74 (urine)	[17]
3	E2BS (E2 binding sites)	Virus	Activation of E6/E7 oncoproteins	Diagnosis of the severity of cervical lesions	Hyper	43 (only HPV-16)	[18]
4	CADM1, MAL, DAPK1	Host	Crucial in cell signaling	Risk of CIN 2/2	Hyper	543 (only HPV 16,18, 31,45)	[19]
5	L1-I, L1-II, L2	Virus	Capsid protein—Immunogenic	Risk of CIN 2/3	Hyper	543 (only HPV 16,18, 31,45)	[19]
6	miR-362-3p (pre-miR-362 promoter)	Host	Controls expression of miR-362-5p/3p	Prognosis of CC	Hyper	31	[20]
7	FAM19A4/ miR124–2	Host		Long-term risk for development of CIN3	Hyper	44,938 (only HPV 16,18)	[21]
8	hsa-miR-124	Host	Tumor suppressing activity	Independent indicator of CIN2+		447	[16]
9	miR-375, miR-196a-1	Host	Deregulation of methylation of miRNAs results in CC		Hyper	30	[22]
10	lncRNA SOX21-AS1		Tumor suppressing activity	Poor prognosis	Hypo	307	[23]

3.2.2 RNA Based Markers

3.2.2.1 miRNA-Based Markers

Around 98% of the human genome consists of non-coding regions, which broadly include micro RNAs (miRNAs), lncRNAs, and circRNAs. miRNAs are around 20 nt long RNAs that can suppress gene expression by binding to the 3'UTR (untranslated region) of miRNAs, which can modulate the expression of close to 60% of coding genes in humans [25]. miRNAs are extremely stable in the sense that they are resistant to ribonucleases in bodily fluids as they exist extracellularly either as exosomes or by forming complexes with proteins such as Ago (Argonaute) [26]. Thus, providing easy accessibility for analysis from bodily fluids. Since a single differentially expressed miRNA may have the same effect in multiple disease conditions, multi-panel miRNA analysis has widely been adopted, further improving the sensitivity and selectivity of the tests [27].

With regard to the use of miRNAs as biomarkers, particularly for CC, they can be broadly classified into the miRNA produced under the influence of HPV genes and others that are not influenced. A study providing evidence for the latter shows that the upregulation of miR-21-5p and downregulation of miR-34a in 118 CC tissue samples analyzed are characteristic of the early onset of CC (pre-neoplastic lesion to CC progression). Particularly, miR-34a shows a significant reduction in expression consistently as the stages of CC progress, starting with CIN1. The human telomerase RNA component (hTERC) reported in the same study is an RNA template for the enzyme telomerase during telomere elongation. While not belonging to the family of miRNA, still being an RNA—has been shown to be found in a significantly higher number of copies as cancer progresses, thus aiding as a marker to identify the transformation of precancerous lesions.

A recent study by Xin Liu shows that the relative overexpression of miR-20a in CC cell lines was facilitated by the HPV E6 gene, which was confirmed based on gene silencing studies. Upon further analysis, it was found that the target for miR-20a—PDCD6 was downregulated, enhancing cell proliferation by activating the Akt/p38 pathway. Thus, providing substantial evidence that the HPV genes can largely influence the miRNA profiles of the host [28] (Fig. 3.2).

However, one of the major challenges concerning the use of miRNA-based biomarkers for the detection of CC includes inconsistencies in results, and thus, universal standardization of protocols in terms of sample collection, analysis, and detection is necessary for greater reliability [30] (Table 3.2).

3.2.2.2 circRNA-Based Markers

Circular RNAs (circRNA) are novel non-coding RNAs that differ from miRNAs, lncRNAs in terms of their structure. Due to the event of back-splicing, the free 5′ and 3′ are joined covalently to form a closed circular structure, unlike their counterparts (miRNA and lncRNA) which are linear [48]. While circRNAs have a variety of mechanisms through which they regulate gene expression, the most critically acclaimed one is their ability to function as miRNA sponges. Every circRNA has miRNA responsive elements (MRE) which can selectively capture miRNAs, acting

Group	N	miR-21-5p expression	miR-34a expression	Percentage of cells with hTERC amplification
Normal or Inflammatory	23	33.90 ± 4.21	20.18 ± 2.23	1.92 ± 1.89
CIN I	42	39.06 ± 4.0	16.46 ± 1.80*	4.99 ± 6.87*
CIN II	20	51.09 ± 7.27*	13.16 ± 1.28*	7.01 ± 5.54*
CIN III	28	65.85 ± 5.56*	10.94 ± 1.24*	12.09 ± 10.32*
SCC	25	104.79 ± 7.44*	9.54 ± 1.26*	24.45 ± 19.84*

Fig. 3.2 Stage dependent expression of various miRNAs as potential biomarkers for CC [29]. (Copyright Received)

like a sponge [49]. The binding of the miRNA to the circRNA results in the disruption of the downstream signaling processes, resulting in aberrant expressions of the sponged miRNAs target [50]. A particularly distinguishing feature of circRNA which aids its applicability as a reliable biomarker among other non-coding is its high stability in mammalian systems and the presence of highly conserved sequences [51]. Their high stability in bodily fluids thus allows detection not only in tissue samples but also in serum, plasma, urine, etc. A list of circRNA-based CC biomarkers reported in the last 3 years has been tabulated in Table 3.3. A few notable studies have been discussed as follows.

An extensive study conducted by Ma et al. on the profiling of circRNA in cervical cancer cell lines revealed that out of a total of 4760 circRNA detected, 9.3% of the circRNAs were differentially expressed in CC cells [59]. Further analysis has provided evidence that the circ_000284 was consistently and significantly overexpressed across five different cervical cell lines under consideration when compared to normal cells. It was concluded that since miR-506 was sponged by circ_000284, it resulted in the overexpression of SNAI1 (Snail—the target of miR-506) which is a protein responsible for the epithelial-to-mesenchymal transition (EMT) facilitating metastasis of carcinoma in situ [62].

While the previously discussed study was pertinent to only in vitro analysis, another study, which included cervical tissue patient samples, suggested the use of circ_0005576 as a potential biomarker for CC. The identified circRNA was a sponge for miR-153-3p and was found to be expressed differentially based on the stage of cancer (CIN1,2a vs CIN2b) and thus was well correlated with the lymph node metastasis status. Based on the Kaplan–Meier regression, it was also concluded that the overall outcome of the patients with high expression of circ_0005576 is poor since the target of miR-153-3p-Kinesin family member 20A (KIF20A) is overexpressed and is known to have excess cell proliferative capacity [63].

However, based on Table 3.3, conclusions have been drawn based on either in vitro models or CC tumor tissue samples. A point to be noted is that in all these reports, the control samples are non-cancerous tissue samples adjacent to the

Table 3.2 List of miRNA-based biomarkers for cervical cancer detection

S. No.	Biomarker	Function of biomarker	Clinical implication	Regulation pattern	Clinical samples	In vitro model	Reference
1	miR-1266	Tumorigenesis	Progression of CC (LSIL to CC)		50 (tissue)		[31]
2	hsa-miR-17-5p, hsa-miR-32-5p, hsa-miR-454-3p		Biosignatures	↑	115 (serum, tissue)		[32]
3	hsa-miR-409-3p		Biosignatures	↓	115 (serum, tissue)		[32]
4	miR-96	Tumor suppressing activity	Progression of CC	↓	83 (tissue)		[33]
5	miR-520d-5p	Tumor suppressing activity	Progression of CC	↓	30 (tissue)		[34]
6	hsa-mir-486-3p, hsa-mir-451a, hsa-mir-144	Oncogenic—Regulates cell growth, apoptosis	Stage dependent expression	↑	248		[35]
7	hsa-mir-424-5p, hsa-mir-450a-2-3p	Tumor suppressing activity	Poor prognosis	↓	248		[35]
8	miR-145	A regulatory gene of RCAN3	Poor prognosis	↓	319		[36]
9	miR-7	Tumor suppressing activity	Poor prognosis	↓		SiHa	[37]
10	miR-149-5p	Tumor suppressing activity	Pathogenesis of HPV	↓	50		[38]
11	miRNA-21, miRNA-20	Oncogenic—Cancer invasion, metastasis	Progression of CC (premalignant to malignant)	↑	80		[39]
12	miRNA-143	Tumor suppressing activity	Progression of CC (temporal)	Premalignant - ↑ CC - ↓	80		[39]
13	miR-1258	Tumor suppressing activity	Progression of CC	↓		SiHa, ca-ski, C33-A	[40]

(continued)

Table 3.2 (continued)

S. No.	Biomarker	Function of biomarker	Clinical implication	Regulation pattern	Clinical samples	In vitro model	Reference
14	miR-409-3p	Tumor suppressing activity—Regulates E6 oncogene activity	Identify the early phase of cervical carcinoma	↓	63		[41]
15	miR-424-5p	Tumor suppressing activity	Progression of CC	↓	29 (tissue)	HeLa, SiHa.	[42]
16	miR-20a	Oncogenic—Invasion, proliferation promoted by HPV 16 E6	Progression of CC	↑		Ca-ski, SiHa	[28]
17	miR-21	Oncogenic—Migration, proliferation by regulating TNF-α	Poor prognosis	↑		HeLa	[43]
18	miR-140-3p	Tumor suppressing activity—Cell cycle arrest, early apoptosis by targeting RRM2	Poor prognosis of cervical cancer	↓		Ca-Ski, C33A, Hela, Hela 229	[44]
19	miR-373-5p	Tumor suppressing activity—Inhibits invasion by targeting FOXC1	Poor prognosis, lymph node metastasis	↓	76		[45]
20	miR-182	Oncogenic—Activated by hr-HPV E7	Stage dependent expression	↑	6 (tissue)	HeLa, SiHa, C33A	[46]
21	miR-449b-5p	Tumor suppressing activity	Poor prognosis	↓	84 (tissue)	HeLa, SiHA, ME180, ca-ski, C33A	[47]
22	miR-21-5p	Oncogenic	Progression of CC (pre-neoplastic lesions to CC)	↑	118 (tissue)		[29]
23	miR-34a	Tumor suppressing activity	Progression of CC (pre-neoplastic lesions to CC)	↓	118 (tissue)		[29]

Table 3.3 List of circRNA-based biomarkers for cervical cancer detection

S. No.	Biomarker	Sponged miRNA	Function of biomarker	Clinical implication	Regulation pattern	Clinical samples	In vitro model	Reference
1	hsa_circ_0007534	miR-498	Oncogenic—Progression of cancer by controlling BMI-1	Progression of CC	↑	45 (tissue)		[52]
2	hsa_circ_0001495		Oncogenic—Regulates epithelial cell proliferation	Tumorigenesis level	↑		RNA sequencing	[53]
3	hsa_circ_0080414		Tumor suppressor—Regulates genes for cervix functioning	Tumorigenesis level	↓		RNA sequencing	[53]
4	hsa_circ_0001445	miR-432	Oncogenic—Proliferation, invasion	Progression of CC	↑	56 (tissue)	HeLa, Ca-Ski, C-33A, SiHa	[54]
5	hsa_circ_0132980	miR-1287-5p	Oncogenic	Progression of CC	↑	35 (tissue)	HT-3, Ca-Ski, C-33A, SiHa	[55]
6	hsa_circ_101996	miR-8075	Oncogenic—Proliferation, migration, invasion	Proportional to the size, stage, lymph node metastasis—Poor prognosis	↑	39 (tissue)	HeLa, Ca-Ski, C-33A, SiHa	[56]
7	hsa_circ_0075341	miR-149-5p	Oncogenic—Proliferation, migration, invasion	Proportional to the size, stage, lymph node metastasis—Poor prognosis	↑	37 (tissue)	SiHa, Ca-Ski	[57]
8	hsa_circ_0004214	miR-485-5p	Oncogenic	Poor prognosis	↑	80 (tissue)	C-33A, HeLa, SiHa, Ca-Ski	[58]
9	hsa_circ_000284	miR-506	Oncogenic—Proliferation, invasion	Poor prognosis	↑		HeLa, CaSki, SiHa, C-33A, SW756	[59]

(continued)

Table 3.3 (continued)

S. No.	Biomarker	Sponged miRNA	Function of biomarker	Clinical implication	Regulation pattern	Clinical samples	In vitro model	Reference
10	hsa_circ_0007874	miR-6893	Oncogenic—Tumorigenesis, chemoresistance	Progression of CC	↑		HeLa, Ca-Ski, C-33A, C-4 II, SiHa	[60]
11	hsa_circ_0005576	miR-153-3p	Oncogenic—Proliferation, motility	Proportional to the stage, lymph node metastasis—Poor prognosis	↑	68 (tissue)	HeLa, Ca-Ski, SiHa, C-33A	[61]

cancerous tissues. Thus, due to variations in gene expression patterns among different tissues (even among adjacent tissues), the results may not be completely reliable. This again raises questions about their abundance in circulating fluids, thus rendering them ineffective in terms of non-invasiveness. Even though circRNAs were discovered in the year 1976, it was not until 2012 that circRNAs in humans were sequenced [64]. Thus, research in the field of circRNAs remains at a primitive stage, requiring further studies to validate their applicability to be used as prognostic biomarkers for CC.

3.2.2.3 lncRNA-Based Markers

Long non-coding RNAs represent 200 nts long non-protein-coding RNAs that lack an open reading frame [65]. In general, lncRNAs regulate cellular processes as transcriptional regulators, recruitment of effectors through scaffold structures, and guide RNAs [66]. In the case of cancer, lncRNAs interfere with normal gene regulation by acting as a miRNA sponge thus affecting downstream signaling pathways, functioning on the same lines as of circRNAs [67]. But unlike circRNAs, they do not consist of highly conserved sequences [68]. The main advantage of the analysis of lncRNAs lies in the fact that there is no need to invasively extract tumor samples for analysis as lncRNAs are stable circulating RNAs and thus their expression can be studied in just the body fluids of patients [69].

A recent list of lncRNA-based markers is tabulated in Table 3.4. A representative study conducted by Duan et al. shows a relatively higher expression of RHPN1 antisense RNA1 (RHPN1-AS1) in CC cell lines in comparison with normal squamous epithelial cells. This has further been substantiated by the analysis of 60 CC tumor tissue samples, which shows a similar trend [75]. Rescue experiments conducted further conclude that the fibroblast growth factor 2 (FGF2) was overexpressed (becoming oncogenic—stem cell-like properties) due to the sponging of miR-299–3p by RHPN1-AS1 thus involved in tumorigenesis by invasion, proliferation, and metastasis of the cancerous cells [77] (Fig. 3.3).

A particularly interesting lncRNA is H19, which has been widely reported to have contradictory roles in the development of CC. While in the case of cell lines, overexpression of H19 (sponging hsa-miR-675) has been observed, but in the case of tissue samples, a lower expression of H19 (miR-138-5p) has been reported [70, 78]. The primary target of miR-675 is involved in controlling the tumor 238 environment and thus facilitates CC migration while miR-138-5p promotes tumor 239 suppression [79, 80]. However, the authors have claimed that the primary cause for the differential miRNA targets is due to stage-dependent molecular alterations in clinical samples which are not profound in cell lines [70].

lncRNAs are a promising candidate to be used as CC biomarkers. However, further research focusing on their practicality is needed since the amount of circulating lncRNAs may not be abundant enough to be sensitively detected. A deeper understanding of the CC stage-dependent release of lncRNAs from the cervical cells into other bodily fluids is essential to extend their applicability in being used as prognostic markers. Most of the differentially expressed lncRNAs are not specific to only CC but are rather found across most cancer types and thus, there is a need to identify highly specific lncRNAs characteristic to only CC.

Table 3.4 List of lncRNA-based biomarkers for cervical cancer detection

S. No.	Biomarker	Sponged miRNA	Function of biomarker	Clinical implication	Regulation pattern	Clinical samples	In vitro model	Reference
1	H19	hsa-miR-675	Modulates key cellular pathways	Poor prognosis	↓	26 (tissue, blood)		[70]
2	PITPNA-AS1	miR-876-5p	Oncogenic—Metastasis, proliferation	Poor prognosis	↑	53 (tissue)		[71]
3	Linc00483	miR-508-3p	Oncogenic—Apoptosis, proliferation, invasion, metastasis	Progression of CC	↑	40 (tissue)	HeLa, SiHa, C-33A, ME 180, ca-ski,	[72]
4	MIR205HG	miR-122-5p	Oncogenic—Progression, regulates cellular processes	Pathogenesis of CC	↑		Ca-ski, MS751, HeLa, SiHa	[73]
5	Lnc-LIF-AS	miR-579-3p, miR-664-3p	Oncogenic—Cell proliferation, migration, invasion	Progression of CC	↑		SiHa, ME-180, C-33A, HeLa	[74]
6	RHPN1-AS1	miR-299-3p	Oncogenic—Tumorigenesis by invasion, proliferation, migration	Progression of CC	↑	60 (tissue)	HeLa, C33A, SiHa	[75]
7	LINC00173	miR-182-5p	Tumor suppressing activity	Poor prognosis	↓	30 (tissue)	HeLa, SiHa, CaSki, C33A	[76]

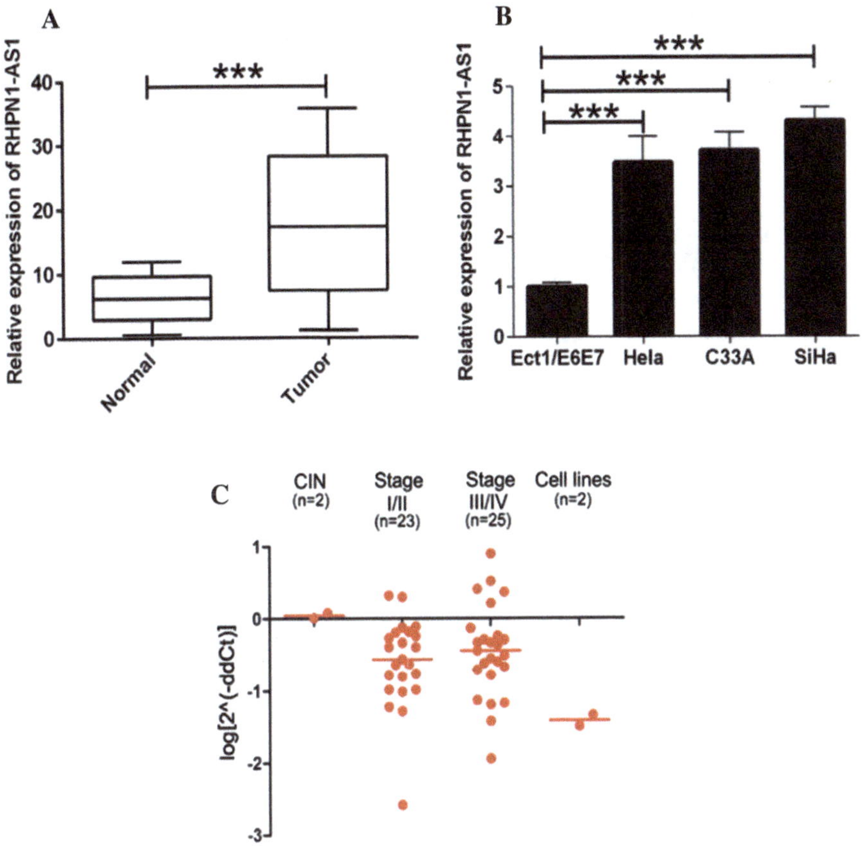

Fig. 3.3 (**a**) CC tissue sample, (**b**) CC cell lines showing significant overexpression of RHPN1-AS1 compared to controls [75]. (**c**) CC stage-dependent downregulation of lnc_H19, [70] in CC cell lines. (Copyrights Received)

3.3 Protein-Based Markers

The protein-based markers are essentially differentially expressed host proteins due to the influence of the HPV oncoproteins. The proteins identified generally play a pivotal role in the cell cycle as it is the tumor-suppressing genes (retinoblastoma—pRb, p53) and proto-oncogenes (EGFR, CDK4, Ras), which are primary targets of the HPV oncoproteins. The following figure (Fig. 3.4) provides an overview of the cell cycle modulations due to the expression of HPV oncogenes E6, E7. As most of these protein-based markers are well established, in the last 3 years, newly identified protein-based markers have been tabulated in Table 3.5.

Since HPV infects the basal cells and moves upwards towards the squamous epithelial cells, it can be ascertained that the topmost or outer layer of the epithelium

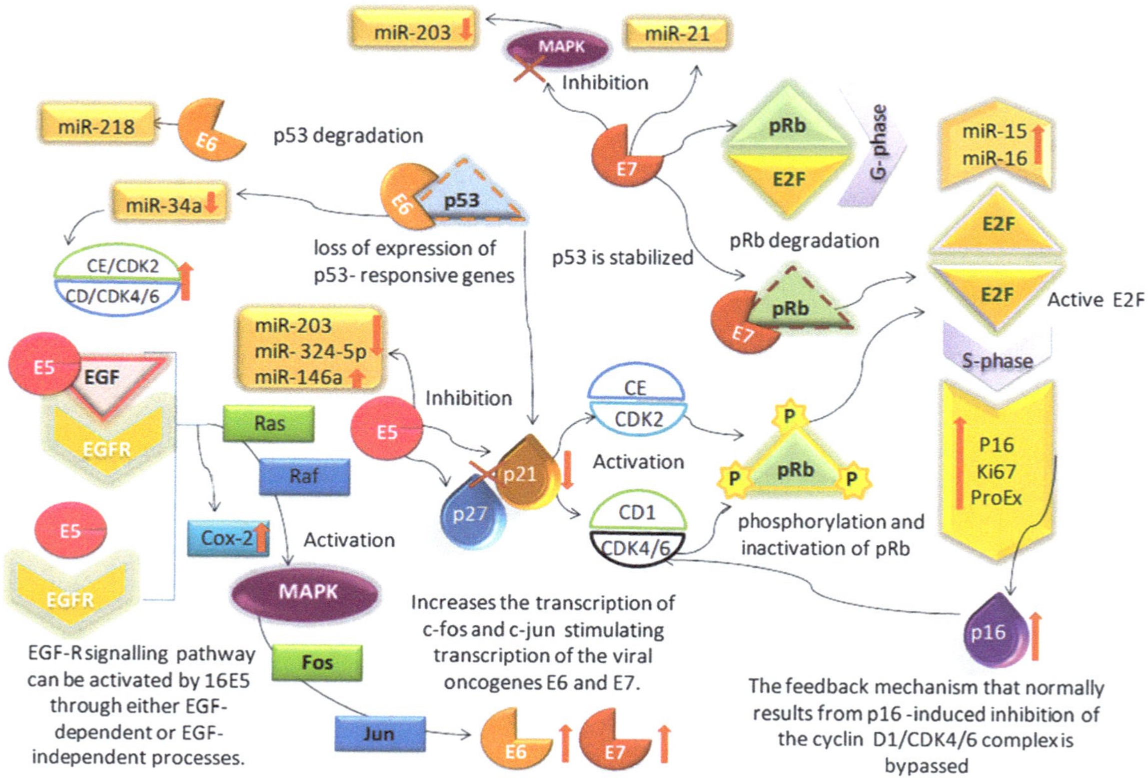

Fig. 3.4 Modulation of cell cycle molecules by HPV oncoproteins [81]. (Copyright Received)

Table 3.5 List of protein-based biomarkers for cervical cancer detection

S. No.	Biomarker	Function of biomarker	Clinical implication	Regulation pattern	Clinical samples	In vitro model	Reference
1	HBXIP	Oncogenic	Progression of CC	↑	107	–	[82]
2	PER1	Maintains cell cycle	Lymph node invasion, stage-dependent expression	↓	248	–	[35]
3	PRKAB1	p53 responsive gene	Stage dependent expression	↓	248	–	[35]
4	PMM2	Glycan synthesis	Lymph node invasion, stage-dependent expression	↓	248	–	[35]
5	RCAN3	A regulatory gene of cellular processes	Poor prognosis	↑	319 (tissue)	–	[36]
6	MTA2	Tumor progression, metastasis	Poor prognosis	↑		SiHa	[37]
7	KLK10	Tumor suppressing activity, regulated by MTA2	Poor prognosis	↓		SiHa	[37]
8	E2F4	Transcription factor, cell cycle regulator	Pathogenesis of HPV	↑	50	–	[38]
9	DTL	Cell cycle regulator, DNA repair	Pathogenesis of HPV	↑	50	–	[38]
10	KIF11	Cell cycle regulator, differentiation, mitosis, MT cross-linking	Pathogenesis of HPV	↑	50	–	[38]
11	SMC4	Oncogene—Proliferation, differentiation, invasion	Pathogenesis of HPV	↑	50	–	[38]
12	RACK1	Activated by HPV E6—Lymphangiogenesis	Poor prognosis	↑	383 (tissue)	HeLa, SiHa, C-33A	[83]
13	SND1	Oncogenic—Proliferation, metastasis, angiogenesis	Poor prognosis	↑	102 (tissue)	Ca-Ski, HeLa, MS-751	[84]
14	hTERC	Telomerase activity	Stage dependent copy number	↑	118 (tissue)	–	[29]
15	CBX7	Tumor suppressing activity	Poor prognosis	↓		HeLa, Ca-Ski	[85]

(exfoliated cervical cells) is a good source to understand the stage of CC. A study by Jin et al. focused on the evaluation of tumor-associated proteins (TAPS) in 146 CC patients' tissue samples based on ELISA. p53, SLeA (Sialyl Lewis A), HPV 16 L1 were identified as potential markers of cervical lesions, while the expression of SLeA in combination with L1 was found to be dependent on the progression of the disease. Also, SLeA and p53 together differentiated CC from normal samples with 91.3% sensitivity and 96.7% specificity [86].

Unlike the other normal protein-based biomarkers correlated to some parts of the aberrant cell signaling pathways of cancerous cells, there are proteins such as the hepatitis B virus X-interacting protein (HBXIP) which have no clearly elucidated mechanism for its role in CC even though its oncogenic role in the development of breast cancer has been well established. The HBXIP overexpression in the study was been found to be inversely proportional to the overall survival rate of patients. Thus, it also serves as a prognostic marker of CC based on immunohistochemical studies on 105 CIN patients when compared to 31 normal cervical epithelial samples. The strongly positive rates of HBXIP expression were close to 57.9% in the case of SCCs and were also found to be strongly correlated with the differentiation stage, p63 expression status (a key player in SCCs tumorigenesis), and lymph node metastasis, as can be concluded from the following figure (Fig. 3.5) [82].

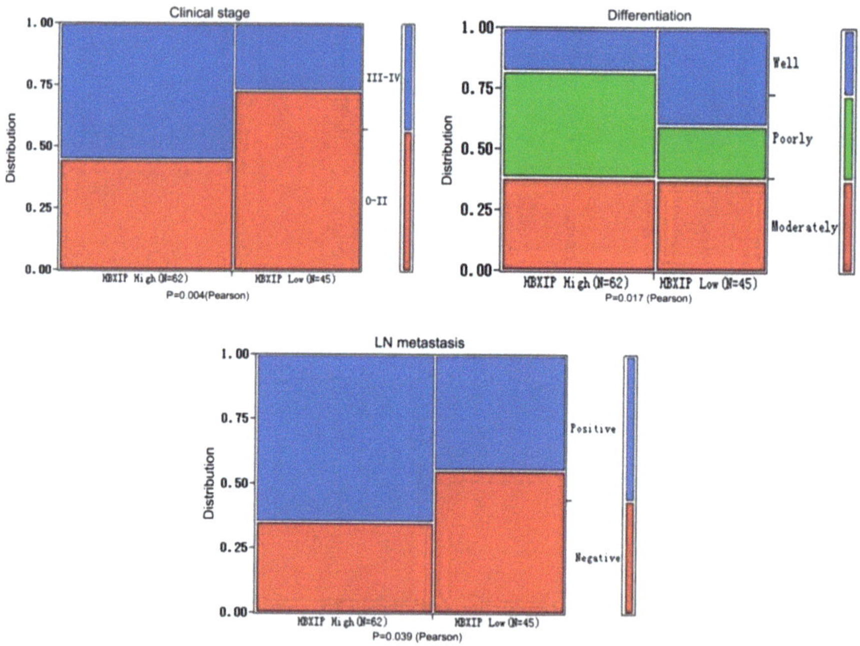

Fig. 3.5 HBXIP overexpression as an indicator of clinical-stage, differentiation, lymph node metastasis of CC [82]. (Copyright Received)

Higher expression of Carcinoembryonic antigen 125 (CA-125), squamous cell carcinoma antigen (SCC-Ag), and highly sensitive C-reactive protein (hs-CRP) in comparison with normal cells has been reported by Guo et al. The authors claim that these protein markers can detect whether recurrence is expected to occur in CC patients. Since the rate of survival is <20% due to the recurrence of that disease within 5 years, this helps improve the treatment time and the survival rate [87].

3.4 Conclusion

Cervical cancer is one of the major causes of morbidity among women. The high morbidity rate is closely associated with the fact that the infection is diagnosed at a very late stage, thus ascertaining the importance of early large-scale screening strategies. While the currently used screening techniques such as cytology have low specificity to detect precancerous lesions, CC biomarkers such as DNA, RNA, protein-based biomarkers have the potential to be exploited for CC diagnosis. While the detection of HPV DNA as a biomarker has been well established, the aspect of epigenetics-based biomarkers has a large potential and so is the case of RNA based biomarkers making them promising candidates for diagnosis and studying the effect of therapy. Further studies in the direction of associating the nucleic acid expression/ methylation patterns with clinical outcomes may provide promising results in terms of disease management with suitable therapeutic interventions. On the other hand, protein-based biomarkers will have to be further studied and validated for their use as CC biomarker as they compromise on specificity unlike the DNA, RNA based markers. Thus, an in-depth evaluation of the molecular and protein-based biomarkers will pave the way to affordable, simple, selective, and specific detection of CC at an early stage.

Declaration of Competing Interest The authors declare no conflicts of interest.

Acknowledgements The authors are grateful to the Ministry of Human Resource Development, Government of India for the financial support through *Scheme for Promotion of Academic and Research Collaboration* (*SPARC*) project "SPARC/2018-2019/P402/SL" We also acknowledge the support received from the National Research Foundation (NRF) of Korea for the Basic Science Research Program funded by the Ministry of Education (NRF-2019R1A6A1A03033215). We are grateful to SASTRA Deemed University, India and SKKU, South Korea for providing infrastructural support.

References

1. Vaccarella S, Laversanne M, Ferlay J, Bray F (2017) Cervical cancer in Africa, Latin America and the Caribbean and Asia: regional inequalities and changing trends. Int J Cancer 141:1997–2001. https://doi.org/10.1002/ijc.30901
2. Biomarkers Definitions Working Group (2001) Biomarkers and surrogate endpoints: preferred definitions and conceptual framework. Clin Pharmacol Ther 69:89–95. https://doi.org/10.1067/mcp.2001.113989

3. Cho HW, So KA, Lee JK, Hong JH (2015) Type-specific persistence or regression of human papillomavirus genotypes in women with cervical intraepithelial neoplasia 1: a prospective cohort study. Obstet Gynecol Sci 58:40–45. https://doi.org/10.5468/ogs.2015.58.1.40
4. Rositch AF, Koshiol J, Hudgens MG, Razzaghi H, Backes DM, Pimenta JM, Franco EL, Poole C, Smith JS (2013) Patterns of persistent genital human papillomavirus infection among women worldwide: a literature review and meta-analysis. Int J Cancer 133:1271–1285. https://doi.org/10.1002/ijc.27828
5. Zur Hausen H (2009) Papillomaviruses in the causation of human cancers — a brief historical account. Virology 384:260–265. https://doi.org/10.1016/j.virol.2008.11.046
6. Cubie HA, Norval M (1988) Synthetic oligonucleotide probes for the detection of human papilloma viruses by in situ hybridisation. J Virol Methods 20:239–249. https://doi.org/10.1016/0166-0934(88)90127-9
7. Cardillo MR, Marino R, Possi V (1991) Human papillomavirus DNA in cervical intraepithelial neoplasia detected by in situ hybridisation. Eur J Cancer Clin Oncol 27:193–197. https://doi.org/10.1016/0277-5379(91)90486-W
8. Ibeanu OA (2011) Molecular pathogenesis of cervical cancer. Cancer Biol Ther 11:295–306. https://doi.org/10.4161/cbt.11.3.14686
9. Wu CT, Morris JR (2001) Genes, genetics, and epigenetics: a correspondence. Science 293:1103 LP–1101105. https://doi.org/10.1126/science.293.5532.1103
10. Dupont C, Armant DR, Brenner CA (2009) Epigenetics: definition, mechanisms and clinical perspective. Semin Reprod Med 27:351–357. https://doi.org/10.1055/s-0029-1237423
11. Jones PA, Baylin SB (2002) The fundamental role of epigenetic events in cancer. Nat Rev Genet 3:415–428. https://doi.org/10.1038/nrg816
12. Graham SV (2010) Human papillomavirus: gene expression, regulation and prospects for novel diagnostic methods and antivrial therapies. Future Microbiol Rev 5:1493–1506. https://doi.org/10.2217/FMB.10.107
13. Bryant D, Onions T, Raybould R, Jones S, Tristram A, Hibbitts S, Fiander A, Powell N (2014) Increased methylation of human papillomavirus type 16 DNA correlates with viral integration in Vulval intraepithelial neoplasia. J Clin Virol 61:393–399. https://doi.org/10.1016/j.jcv.2014.08.006
14. Szalmás A, Kónya J (2009) Epigenetic alterations in cervical carcinogenesis. Semin Cancer Biol 19:144–152. https://doi.org/10.1016/j.semcancer.2009.02.011
15. Chaiwongkot A, Niruthisard S, Kitkumthorn N, Bhattarakosol P (2017) Quantitative methylation analysis of human papillomavirus 16 L1 gene reveals potential biomarker for cervical cancer progression. Diagn Microbiol Infect Dis 89:265–270. https://doi.org/10.1016/j.diagmicrobio.2017.08.010
16. Rogeri CD, Silveira HCS, Causin RL, Villa LL, Stein MD, de Carvalho AC, Arantes LMRB, Scapulatempo-Neto C, Possati-Resende JC, Antoniazzi M et al (2018) Methylation of the hsa-miR-124, SOX1, TERT, and LMX1A genes as biomarkers for precursor lesions in cervical cancer. Gynecol Oncol 150:545–551. https://doi.org/10.1016/j.ygyno.2018.06.014
17. van den Helder R, van Trommel NE, van Splunter AP, Lissenberg-Witte BI, Bleeker MCG, Steenbergen RDM (2020) Methylation analysis in urine fractions for optimal CIN3 and cervical cancer detection. Papillomavirus Res 9:100193. https://doi.org/10.1016/j.pvr.2020.100193
18. Zhang X, Zhi Y, Li Y, Fan T, Li H, Du P, Cheng G, Li X (2019) Study on the relationship between methylation status of HPV 16 E2 binding sites and cervical lesions. Clin Chim Acta 493:98–103. https://doi.org/10.1016/j.cca.2019.02.027
19. Fiano V, Trevisan M, Fasanelli F, Grasso C, Marabese F, da Graça Bicalho M, de Carvalho NS, Maestri CA, Merletti F, Sacerdote C et al (2018) Methylation in host and viral genes as marker of aggressiveness in cervical lesions: analysis in 543 unscreened women. Gynecol Oncol 151:319–326. https://doi.org/10.1016/j.ygyno.2018.08.031
20. Song L, Liu S, Yao H, Zhang L, Li Y, Xu D, Li Q (2019) MiR-362-3p is downregulated by promoter methylation and independently predicts shorter OS of cervical squamous cell carcinoma. Biomed Pharmacother 115:108944. https://doi.org/10.1016/j.biopha.2019.108944

21. Dick S, Kremer WW, De Strooper LMA, Lissenberg-Witte BI, Steenbergen RDM, Meijer CJLM, Berkhof J, Heideman DAM (2019) Long-term CIN3+ risk of HPV positive women after triage with FAM19A4/miR124-2 methylation analysis. Gynecol Oncol 154:368–373. https://doi.org/10.1016/j.ygyno.2019.06.002
22. Varghese VK, Shukla V, Jishnu PV, Kabekkodu SP, Pandey D, Sharan K, Satyamoorthy K (2019) Characterizing methylation regulated miRNA in carcinoma of the human uterine cervix. Life Sci 232:116668. https://doi.org/10.1016/j.lfs.2019.116668
23. Wang R, Li Y, Du P, Zhang X, Li X, Cheng G (2019) Hypomethylation of the lncRNA SOX21-AS1 has clinical prognostic value in cervical cancer. Life Sci:233. https://doi.org/10.1016/j.lfs.2019.116708
24. Lorincz AT (2011) The promise and the problems of epigenetics biomarkers in cancer. Expert Opin Med Diagn 5:375–379. https://doi.org/10.1517/17530059.2011.590129
25. O'Brien J, Hayder H, Zayed Y, Peng C (2018) Overview of MicroRNA biogenesis, mechanisms of actions, and circulation. Front Endocrinol (Lausanne) 9:402. https://doi.org/10.3389/fendo.2018.00402
26. Arroyo JD, Chevillet JR, Kroh EM, Ruf IK, Pritchard CC, Gibson DF, Mitchell PS, Bennett CF, Pogosova-Agadjanyan EL, Stirewalt DL et al (2011) Argonaute2 complexes carry a population of circulating microRNAs independent of vesicles in human plasma. Proc Natl Acad Sci U S A 108:5003–5008. https://doi.org/10.1073/pnas.1019055108
27. Condrat CE, Thompson DC, Barbu MG, Bugnar OL, Boboc A, Cretoiu D, Suciu N, Cretoiu SM, Voinea SC (2020) miRNAs as biomarkers in disease: latest findings regarding their role in diagnosis and prognosis. Cell 9:276. https://doi.org/10.3390/cells9020276
28. Liu X (2018) Up-regulation of miR-20a by HPV16 E6 exerts growth-promoting effects by targeting PDCD6 in cervical carcinoma cells. Biomed Pharmacother 102:996–1002. https://doi.org/10.1016/j.biopha.2018.03.154
29. Zhu Y, Han Y, Tian T, Su P, Jin G, Chen J, Cao Y (2018) MiR-21-5p, miR-34a, and human telomerase RNA component as surrogate markers for cervical cancer progression. Pathol Res Pract 214:374–379. https://doi.org/10.1016/j.prp.2018.01.001
30. Chevillet JR, Lee I, Briggs HA, He Y, Wang K (2014) Issues and prospects of microRNA-based biomarkers in blood and other body fluids. Molecules 19:6080–6105. https://doi.org/10.3390/molecules19056080
31. Wang J, Liu Y, Wang X, Li J, Wei J, Wang Y, Song W, Zhang Z (1864) MiR-1266 promotes cell proliferation, migration and invasion in cervical cancer by targeting DAB2IP. Biochim Biophys Acta Mol basis Dis 2018:3623–3630. https://doi.org/10.1016/j.bbadis.2018.09.028
32. Shukla V, Varghese VK, Kabekkodu SP, Mallya S, Chakrabarty S, Jayaram P, Pandey D, Banerjee S, Sharan K, Satyamoorthy K (2019) Enumeration of deregulated miRNAs in liquid and tissue biopsies of cervical cancer. Gynecol Oncol 155:135–143. https://doi.org/10.1016/j.ygyno.2019.08.012
33. Yang L, Liu L, Zhang X, Zhu Y, Li L, Wang B, Liu Y, Ren C (2020) miR-96 enhances the proliferation of cervical cancer cells by targeting FOXO1. Pathol Res Pract 216:152854. https://doi.org/10.1016/j.prp.2020.152854
34. Zhang L, Liu F, Fu Y, Chen X, Zhang D (2020) MiR-520d-5p functions as a tumor-suppressor gene in cervical cancer through targeting PTK2. Life Sci 254:117558. https://doi.org/10.1016/j.lfs.2020.117558
35. Yang C, Ren J, Li B, Zhang D, Ma C, Cheng C, Sun Y, Fu L, Shi X (2018) Identification of clinical tumor stages related mRNAs and miRNAs in cervical squamous cell carcinoma. Pathol Res Pract 214:1638–1647. https://doi.org/10.1016/j.prp.2018.07.035
36. Zhang XY, Ma H, Li J, Lu XR, Li JQ, Yuan N, Zhang ZL, Xue XY (2020) Functional implications of miR-145/RCAN3 axis in the progression of cervical cancer. Reprod Biol 20:140–146. https://doi.org/10.1016/j.repbio.2020.04.001
37. Lin CL, Ying TH, Yang SF, Wang SW, Cheng SP, Lee JJ, Hsieh YH (2020) Transcriptional suppression of miR-7 by MTA2 induces Sp1-mediated KLK10 expression and metastasis of

cervical cancer. Mol Ther Nucleic Acids 20:699–710. https://doi.org/10.1016/j.omtn.2020.04.009

38. Yuan Y, Shi X, Li B, Peng M, Zhu T, Lv G, Liu L, Jin H, Li L, Qin D (2020) Integrated analysis of key microRNAs /TFs /mRNAs/ in HPV-positive cervical cancer based on microRNA sequencing and bioinformatics analysis. Pathol Res Pract 216:152952. https://doi.org/10.1016/j.prp.2020.152952
39. Jihad NA, Naif HM (2020) Evaluation of microRNA-20, −21 and −143 expression in human papilloma virus induced premalignant and malignant cervical lesions. Gene Rep 20:100702. https://doi.org/10.1016/j.genrep.2020.100702
40. Peng X, Zhang Y, Gao J, Cai C (2020) MiR-1258 promotes the apoptosis of cervical cancer cells by regulating the E2F1/P53 signaling pathway. Exp Mol Pathol 114:104368. https://doi.org/10.1016/j.yexmp.2020.104368
41. Sommerova L, Anton M, Bouchalova P, Jasickova H, Rak V, Jandakova E, Selingerova I, Bartosik M, Vojtesek B, Hrstka R (2019) The role of miR-409-3p in regulation of HPV16/18-E6 mRNA in human cervical high-grade squamous intraepithelial lesions. Antivir Res 163:185–192. https://doi.org/10.1016/j.antiviral.2019.01.019
42. Zhou Y, An Q, Xia Guo R, Huan Qiao Y, Xia Li L, Yan Zhang X, Zhao X (2017) Lan miR424-5p functions as an anti-oncogene in cervical cancer cell growth by targeting KDM5B via the notch signaling pathway. Life Sci 171:9–15. https://doi.org/10.1016/j.lfs.2017.01.006
43. Xu L, Xu Q, Li X, Zhang X (2017) MicroRNA-21 regulates the proliferation and apoptosis of cervical cancer cells via tumor necrosis factor-α. Mol Med Rep 16:4659–4663. https://doi.org/10.3892/mmr.2017.7143
44. Ma J, Zhang F, Sun P (2020) miR-140-3p impedes the proliferation of human cervical cancer cells by targeting RRM2 to induce cell-cycle arrest and early apoptosis. Bioorganic Med Chem 28:115283. https://doi.org/10.1016/j.bmc.2019.115283
45. Huang Y, Huang H, Li M, Zhang X, Liu Y, Wang Y (2017) MicroRNA-374c-5p regulates the invasion and migration of cervical cancer by acting on the Foxc1/snail pathway. Biomed Pharmacother 94:1038–1047. https://doi.org/10.1016/j.biopha.2017.07.150
46. Chen J, Deng Y, Ao L, Song Y, Xu Y, Wang CC, Choy KW, Tony Chung KH, Du Q, Sui Y et al (2019) The high-risk HPV oncogene E7 upregulates miR-182 expression through the TGF-β/Smad pathway in cervical cancer. Cancer Lett 460:75–85. https://doi.org/10.1016/j.canlet.2019.06.015
47. Cheng L, Shi X, Huo D, Zhao Y, Zhang H (2019) MiR-449b-5p regulates cell proliferation, migration and radioresistance in cervical cancer by interacting with the transcription suppressor FOXP1. Eur J Pharmacol 856:172399. https://doi.org/10.1016/j.ejphar.2019.05.028
48. Memczak S, Jens M, Elefsinioti A, Torti F, Krueger J, Rybak A, Maier L, Mackowiak SD, Gregersen LH, Munschauer M (2013) Circular RNAs are a large class of animal RNAs with regulatory potency. Nature 495:333–338
49. Tay Y, Rinn J, Pandolfi PP (2014) The multilayered complexity of ceRNA crosstalk and competition. Nature 505:344–352
50. Hansen TB, Wiklund ED, Bramsen JB, Villadsen SB, Statham AL, Clark SJ, Kjems J (2011) miRNA-dependent gene silencing involving Ago2-mediated cleavage of a circular antisense RNA. EMBO J 30:4414–4422. https://doi.org/10.1038/emboj.2011.359
51. Hansen TB, Jensen TI, Clausen BH, Bramsen JB, Finsen B, Damgaard CK, Kjems J (2013) Natural RNA circles function as efficient microRNA sponges. Nature 495:384–388. https://doi.org/10.1038/nature11993
52. Rong X, Gao W, Yang X, Guo J (2019) Downregulation of hsa_circ_0007534 restricts the proliferation and invasion of cervical cancer through regulating miR-498/BMI-1 signaling. Life Sci 235:116785. https://doi.org/10.1016/j.lfs.2019.116785
53. Huang H, Chen YF, Du X, Zhang C (2020) Identification and characterization of tumorigenic circular RNAs in cervical cancer. Cell Signal 73:109669. https://doi.org/10.1016/j.cellsig.2020.109669

54. Huang P, Qi B, Yao H, Zhang L, Li Y, Li Q (2020) Circular RNA cSMARCA5 regulates the progression of cervical cancer by acting as a microRNA-432 sponge. Mol Med Rep 21:1217–1223. https://doi.org/10.3892/mmr.2020.10910
55. Ji F, Du R, Chen T, Zhang M, Zhu Y, Luo X, Ding Y (2020) Circular RNA circSLC26A4 accelerates cervical cancer progression via miR-1287-5p/HOXA7 Axis. Mol Ther Nucleic Acids 19:413–420. https://doi.org/10.1016/j.omtn.2019.11.032
56. Song T, Xu A, Zhang Z, Gao F, Zhao L, Chen X, Gao J, Kong X (2019) CircRNA hsa_circRNA_101996 increases cervical cancer proliferation and invasion through activating TPX2 expression by restraining miR-8075. J Cell Physiol 234:14296–14305. https://doi.org/10.1002/jcp.28128
57. Shao S, Wang C, Wang S, Zhang H, Zhang Y (2020) Hsa_circ_0075341 is up-regulated and exerts oncogenic properties by sponging miR-149-5p in cervical cancer. Biomed Pharmacother 121:109582. https://doi.org/10.1016/j.biopha.2019.109582
58. Ou R, Lv J, Zhang Q, Lin F, Zhu L, Huang F, Li X, Li T, Zhao L, Ren Y et al (2020) circAMOTL1 motivates AMOTL1 expression to facilitate cervical cancer growth. Mol Ther Nucleic Acids 19:50–60. https://doi.org/10.1016/j.omtn.2019.09.022
59. Ma HB, Yao YN, Yu JJ, Chen XX, Li HF (2018) Extensive profiling of circular RNAs and the potential regulatory role of circRNA-000284 in cell proliferation and invasion of cervical cancer via sponging miR-506. Am J Transl Res 10:592–604
60. Chen M, Ai G, Zhou J, Mao W, Li H, Guo J (2019) circMTO1 promotes tumorigenesis and chemoresistance of cervical cancer via regulating miR-6893. Biomed Pharmacother 117:109064. https://doi.org/10.1016/j.biopha.2019.109064
61. Ma H, Tian T, Liu X, Xia M, Chen C, Mai L, Xie S, Yu L (2019) Upregulated circ_0005576 facilitates cervical cancer progression via the miR-153/KIF20A axis. Biomed Pharmacother 118. https://doi.org/10.1016/j.biopha.2019.109311
62. Bolós V, Peinado H, Pérez-Moreno MA, Fraga MF, Esteller M, Cano A (2003) The transcription factor slug represses E-cadherin expression and induces epithelial to mesenchymal transitions: a comparison with snail and E47 repressors. J Cell Sci 116:499–511
63. Gasnereau I, Boissan M, Margall-ducos G, Couchy G, Wendum D, Bourgain-guglielmetti F, Desdouets C, Lacombe M (2012) KIF20A mRNA and its product MKlp2 are increased during hepatocyte proliferation and Hepatocarcinogenesis. Am J Pathol 180:131–140. https://doi.org/10.1016/j.ajpath.2011.09.040
64. Sanger HL, Klotz G, Riesner D, Gross HJ, Kleinschmidt AK (1976) Viroids are single-stranded covalently closed circular RNA molecules existing as highly base-paired rod-like structures. Proc Natl Acad Sci 73:3852 LP–3853856. https://doi.org/10.1073/pnas.73.11.3852
65. Mattick JS (2001) Non-coding RNAs: the architects of eukaryotic complexity. EMBO Rep 2:986–991. https://doi.org/10.1093/embo-reports/kve230
66. Zhang H, Chen Z, Wang X, Huang Z, He Z, Chen Y (2013) Long non-coding RNA: a new player in cancer. J Hematol Oncol 6:37. https://doi.org/10.1186/1756-8722-6-37
67. Cheetham SW, Gruhl F, Mattick JS, Dinger ME (2013) Long noncoding RNAs and the genetics of cancer. Br J Cancer 108:2419–2425. https://doi.org/10.1038/bjc.2013.233
68. Necsulea A, Soumillon M, Warnefors M, Liechti A, Daish T, Zeller U, Baker JC, Grützner F, Kaessmann H (2014) The evolution of lncRNA repertoires and expression patterns in tetrapods. Nature 505:635–640. https://doi.org/10.1038/nature12943
69. Shi T, Gao G, Cao Y (2016) Long noncoding RNAs as novel biomarkers have a promising future in cancer diagnostics. Dis Markers 2016:9085195. https://doi.org/10.1155/2016/9085195
70. Roychowdhury A, Samadder S, Das P, Mazumder DI, Chatterjee A, Addya S, Mondal R, Roy A, Roychoudhury S, Panda CK (2020) Deregulation of H19 is associated with cervical carcinoma. Genomics 112:961–970. https://doi.org/10.1016/j.ygeno.2019.06.012
71. Guo Q, Li L, Bo Q, Chen L, Sun L, Shi H (2020) Long noncoding RNA PITPNA-AS1 promotes cervical cancer progression through regulating the cell cycle and apoptosis by

targeting the miR-876-5p/c-MET axis. Biomed Pharmacother 128:1–10. https://doi.org/10.1016/j.biopha.2020.110072
72. Hu P, Zhou G, Zhang X, Song G, Zhan L, Cao Y (2019) Long non-coding RNA Linc00483 accelerated tumorigenesis of cervical cancer by regulating miR-508-3p/RGS17 axis. Life Sci 234:116789. https://doi.org/10.1016/j.lfs.2019.116789
73. Dong M, Dong Z, Zhu X, Zhang Y, Song L (2019) Long non-coding RNA MIR205HG regulates KRT17 and tumor processes in cervical cancer via interaction with SRSF1. Exp Mol Pathol 111:104322. https://doi.org/10.1016/j.yexmp.2019.104322
74. Song W, Wang J, Liu H, Zhu C, Xu F, Qian L, Shen Z, Zhu J, Yin S, Qin J et al (2019) Effects of LncRNA Lnc-LIF-AS on cell proliferation, migration and invasion in a human cervical cancer cell line. Cytokine 120:165–175. https://doi.org/10.1016/j.cyto.2019.05.004
75. Duan H, Li X, Chen Y, Wang Y, Li Z (2019) LncRNA RHPN1-AS1 promoted cell proliferation, invasion and migration in cervical cancer via the modulation of miR-299–3p/FGF2 axis. Life Sci 239:116856. https://doi.org/10.1016/j.lfs.2019.116856
76. Zhang J, Zhou M, Zhao X, Wang G, Li J (2020) Long noncoding RNA LINC00173 is downregulated in cervical cancer and inhibits cell proliferation and invasion by modulating the miR-182-5p/FBXW7 axis. Pathol Res Pract 216:152994. https://doi.org/10.1016/j.prp.2020.152994
77. Song K-H, Cho H, Kim S, Lee H-J, Oh SJ, Woo SR, Hong S-O, Jang HS, Noh KH, Choi CH et al (2017) API5 confers cancer stem cell-like properties through the FGF2-NANOG axis. Oncogenesis 6:e285–e285. https://doi.org/10.1038/oncsis.2016.87
78. Ou L, Wang D, Zhang H, Yu Q, Hua F (2018) Decreased expression of miR-138-5p by lncRNA H19 in cervical cancer promotes tumor proliferation. Oncol Res 26:401–410. https://doi.org/10.3727/096504017X15017209042610
79. Raveh E, Matouk IJ, Gilon M, Hochberg A (2015) The H19 long non-coding RNA in cancer initiation, progression and metastasis - a proposed unifying theory. Mol Cancer 14:184. https://doi.org/10.1186/s12943-015-0458-2
80. Yeh M, Oh CS, Yoo JY, Kaur B, Lee TJ (2019) Pivotal role of microRNA-138 in human cancers. Am J Cancer Res 9:1118–1126
81. De Freitas AC, Coimbra EC, da Leitão MCG (2014) Molecular targets of HPV oncoproteins: potential biomarkers for cervical carcinogenesis. Biochim Biophys Acta - Rev Cancer 1845:91–103. https://doi.org/10.1016/j.bbcan.2013.12.004
82. Li N, Wang Y, Che S, Yang Y, Piao J, Liu S, Lin Z (2017) HBXIP over expression as an independent biomarker for cervical cancer. Exp Mol Pathol 102:133–137. https://doi.org/10.1016/j.yexmp.2017.01.009
83. Wu H, Song S, Yan A, Guo X, Chang L, Xu L, Hu L, Kuang M, Liu B, He D et al (2020) RACK1 promotes the invasive activities and lymph node metastasis of cervical cancer via galectin-1. Cancer Lett 469:287–300. https://doi.org/10.1016/j.canlet.2019.11.002
84. Zhan F, Zhong Y, Qin Y, Li L, Wu W, Yao M (2020) SND1 facilitates the invasion and migration of cervical cancer cells by Smurf1-mediated degradation of FOXA2. Exp Cell Res 388:111809. https://doi.org/10.1016/j.yexcr.2019.111809
85. Li R, Yan Q, Tian P, Wang Y, Wang J, Tao N, Ning L, Lin X, Ding L, Liu J et al (2019) CBX7 inhibits cell growth and motility and induces apoptosis in cervical cancer cells. Mol Ther - Oncolytics 15:108–116. https://doi.org/10.1016/j.omto.2019.09.002
86. Jin Y, Kim SC, Kim HJ, Ju W, Kim YH, Kim HJ (2018) Use of protein-based biomarkers of exfoliated cervical cells for primary screening of cervical cancer. Arch Pharm Res 41:438–449. https://doi.org/10.1007/s12272-018-1015-5
87. Guo S, Yang B, Liu H, Li Y, Li S, Ma L, Liu J, Guo W (2017) Serum expression level of squamous cell carcinoma antigen, highly sensitive C-reactive protein, and CA-125 as potential biomarkers for recurrence of cervical cancer. J Cancer Res Ther 13:689–692. https://doi.org/10.4103/jcrt.JCRT_414_17

Methods for Screening of Cervical Cancer: State of Art

4

Shrute Kannappan, Jung Heon Lee, and
John Bosco Balaguru Rayappan

Abstract

Only 1% of HPV infected patients show visible warts or condylomas. Thence, diagnosis of cervical cancer requires other techniques to identify the internal lesions. Traditional methods for the detection of HPV include cytology-based methods, serological methods and nucleic acid-based methods. The cytology-based methods are the papanicolaou (Pap) smear test and visual inspection with acetic acid (VIA). As these microscopy-based methods cannot differentiate between the type of HPV (high, intermediate or low risk), molecular techniques such as serological detection (detection of serum antibodies produced

S. Kannappan
Department of Molecular Cell Biology, School of Medicine, Sungkyunkwan University (SKKU), Suwon, South Korea

Research Center for Advanced Materials Technology, Sungkyunkwan University (SKKU), Suwon, South Korea

J. H. Lee (✉)
School of Advanced Materials Science and Engineering, Research Center for Advanced Materials Technology, Biomedical Institute for Convergence at SKKU (BICS), Sungkyunkwan University (SKKU), Suwon, Republic of Korea

School of Advanced Materials Science & Engineering, Sungkyunkwan University (SKKU), Suwon, South Korea

Biomedical Institute for Convergence at SKKU (BICS), Sungkyunkwan University (SKKU), Suwon, South Korea
e-mail: jhlee7@skku.edu

J. B. B. Rayappan
Centre for Nanotechnology and Advanced Biomaterials (CeNTAB), School of Electrical and Electronics Engineering, SASTRA Deemed University, Thanjavur, Tamil Nadu, India

J. B. B. Rayappan, J. H. Lee (eds.), *Biomarkers and Biosensors for Cervical Cancer Diagnosis*, https://doi.org/10.1007/978-981-16-2586-2_4

as a result of the humoral immune response against the viral infection), in situ hybridization, southern blotting and dot blotting were adopted. Owing to the low sensitivity of the methods formerly stated and need for large amounts of DNA, nucleic acid-based amplification techniques such as PCR (polymerase chain reaction), microarray and next generation sequencing (NGS) are being adopted currently. A few U.S. Food and Drug Administration (FDA)-approved commercial HPV testing kits include the Qiagen Hybrid Capture 2 High-Risk HPV DNA Test, Cervista HPV 16/18 Genotyping Test, Cobas HPV Assay and Aptima HPV Assay, which are all solely based on nucleic acid-based detection. These methods, however, are not affordable for large-scale screening due to expensive instrumentation and analysis systems, limited specificity and sensitivity. Thus, rapid testing in modular units, establishment of universal standards to test the analytical efficiency of the different tests based on large-scale clinical trials and affordability are aspects of the HPV test kits, which need to be improved upon to develop globally usable point-of-care testing systems.

Keywords

Cobas · Aptima · Cervista · HPV test · Cervical cancer test

4.1 Introduction

In general, cancer screening is dependent on the organ suspected to have an uncontrolled growth of cells. Screening techniques for the most common types of cancer include mammography for breast cancer [1], colonoscopy for colon cancer [2], alpha-fetoprotein-based blood test for liver cancer [3], CT scan for lung cancer [4], etc. Unlike the aforementioned types of cancers, cervical cancer (CC) is unique in the sense that it is caused by a viral infection. Thus, the primary aim of CC screening tests is to detect the presence of a viral infection. Only 1% of patients infected with HPV show visible warts or condylomas, limiting diagnosis by visual examination [5]. Diagnosis of CC in asymptomatic patients thus requires other techniques to identify the presence of the virus itself. Thus, the general strategies to detect viruses include antibody tests, viral antigen detection tests, viral culture tests and nucleic acid-based tests [6]. While thc serology-based techniques (antigen, antibody detection) have limited specificity, viral culture tests are particularly not suitable for HPV detection since it cannot be propagated using conventional cell culture techniques as cell differentiation is required for the completion of the viral replication cycle [7]. However, a traditionally developed alternative for screening CC was the cytological examination of cervical smears. In recent days, the most common method to detect HPV infection is the nucleic acid-based methods [8].

4.2 Cytology-Based Methods

Over the last 75 years, the Papanicolaou test developed by Georgios Papanikolaou has been the primary test for screening CC [9]. The basic principle of the Pap test is to microscopically detect precancerous/cancerous lesions in exfoliated cervical cells stained with the Pap reagent [10]. The cervical cell specimens are collected by inserting and rotating a swab or brush into the cervix and are either directly transferred to a microscope slide for examination or are resuspended in an appropriate medium for further analysis (liquid-based cytology) [11]. Upon examination, the cytologists classify the samples based on the Bethesda classification and refer the patients either for colposcopy or repeat cytology if abnormalities such as the presence of koilocytes (nuclear enlargements, hyperchromasia, perinuclear halo), which are hallmarks for a productive HPV infection, are observed [12]. Colposcopy is generally not preferred since patients experience several side effects due to the localized distress caused by the visual examination of the cervix using a colposcope [13]. Besides, it is a rather expensive and time-consuming procedure with relatively lower sensitivity in the case of invasive carcinoma [14]. Thus, the Pap test is considered as a primary screening technique for the detection of CC.

However, one of the major limitations of the Pap smear test is that there is a higher probability of false negatives since, unlike serological and nucleic acid tests, which provide a quantitative measure, serological tests are rather qualitative. Thence, there is variability in the interpretation of samples depending on the technician's expertise. Also, visual examination only allows one to conclude the presence of lesions but does not ascertain the specific subtype of HPV (typing) behind the infection. Thus, a nucleic acid-based test for typing the HPV causing the infection is invariably necessary to predict the prognosis of the patient and start with suitable intervention.

An alternative technique in place of the Pap smear test is the visual inspection of the cervix with acetic acid (VIA). The examination is conducted by applying a 3–5% solution of acetic acid to the uterine cervix and looking for the appearance of white colour. In the presence of excessive proteins, the tissue turns white, which is a characteristic feature of a precancerous lesion as the acetic acid coagulates the proteins resulting in white colour [15]. A similar test performed after VIA is VILI—Visual inspection with Lugol's Iodine, which stains glycogen in black colour while the absence of glycogen in the tissue is signified by a yellow colour. Since the precancerous lesions lack glycogen, the presence of an HPV infection with a high probability of progressing into cervical carcinoma is characterized by the appearance of a yellow colour [16]. These tests are generally used in combination with the Pap smear test particularly in case the lesions are difficult to identify visually. While electron microscopy offers a viable option to visually examine for the presence of the virus, it cannot detect the presence of a precancerous lesion and limits the ability to perform HPV typing. Similar to the Pap smear test, VIA and VILI also suffer from the same limitations. To compensate for the poor sensitivity of the Pap smear test (50–80%), repeated Pap smear testing is generally performed given the ease of performing the test [17].

4.3 Serological Methods

With the advent of molecular techniques, detection of serum antibodies produced as a result of the humoral immune response against viral infection through techniques such as ELISA (Enzyme-linked immunosorbent assay) [18], western blot [19], RIA (radioimmunoassay) [20] has been adopted. The anti-L1 antibody is one such antibody that is characteristic of an HPV infection, however, is independent of the type of cancer [21]. On the other hand, the presence of an anti-E7 antibody is a hallmark of CC caused by an HPV infection with up to 80% prevalence in clinical samples [22]. Since L1 is a late structural protein expressed at a relatively later stage of CC, this immunocytochemistry-based technique is rather ineffective in identifying precancerous lesions at an early stage and suffers from low sensitivity.

4.4 Nucleic Acid-Based Methods

Southern blot was one of the first molecular techniques to detect HPV DNA in clinical samples, after DNA isolation and restriction digestion [23]. A modified version of the southern blot is the dot blot where the specimen is directly spotted onto a membrane, unlike the former, where the sample is transferred from a gel to a blotting membrane and further analysed [24]. Further, filter-based in situ hybridization has emerged as one of the pioneering techniques to detect HPV DNA directly in the clinical samples and can be strongly correlated to its histology [25]. The spatial location of the viral genome (integrated or episomal) can be ascertained, thus correlating with the probability of the infection progressing into invasive carcinoma. The clinical samples used in both the cases must be highly preserved to prevent DNA degradation failing, which may result in false-negative results. Since the limit of detection for southern blot (100,000 copies per test) and in situ hybridization (25 copies of HPV DNA per cell) is not sufficiently low, it fails to effectively detect high-grade lesions without prior DNA amplification of the samples [26]. In addition, both techniques are time-consuming, highly sensitive to minor changes in the experimental protocol and require a wide array of radioactive probes for genotyping, increasing the risk of cross-reactivity.

As of 2015, there are currently 193 different commercially available HPV test kits [27]. The following section will briefly elaborate on a few FDA approved HPV tests, which are currently used for HPV testing. One of the first PCR free HPV detection kits approved by the FDA in 2003 is the Hybrid Capture 2 (HC2) kit, which can identify the presence of 18 different types of HPV (13 high risk-HPV (hr-HPV), 5 low risk-HPV (lr-HPV)) using a combination of capture RNA, capture antibodies and enzymatic reactions as described in the following Fig. 4.1a [28]. Since the assay is designed in such a way that more than one antibody can bind to a given DNA–RNA hybrid, it aids in signal amplification, resulting in a readout by a luminometer in terms of relative luminescence unit (RLU) depending on the presence of HPV DNA in the sample under consideration. The test kit allows for high throughput screening as currently,

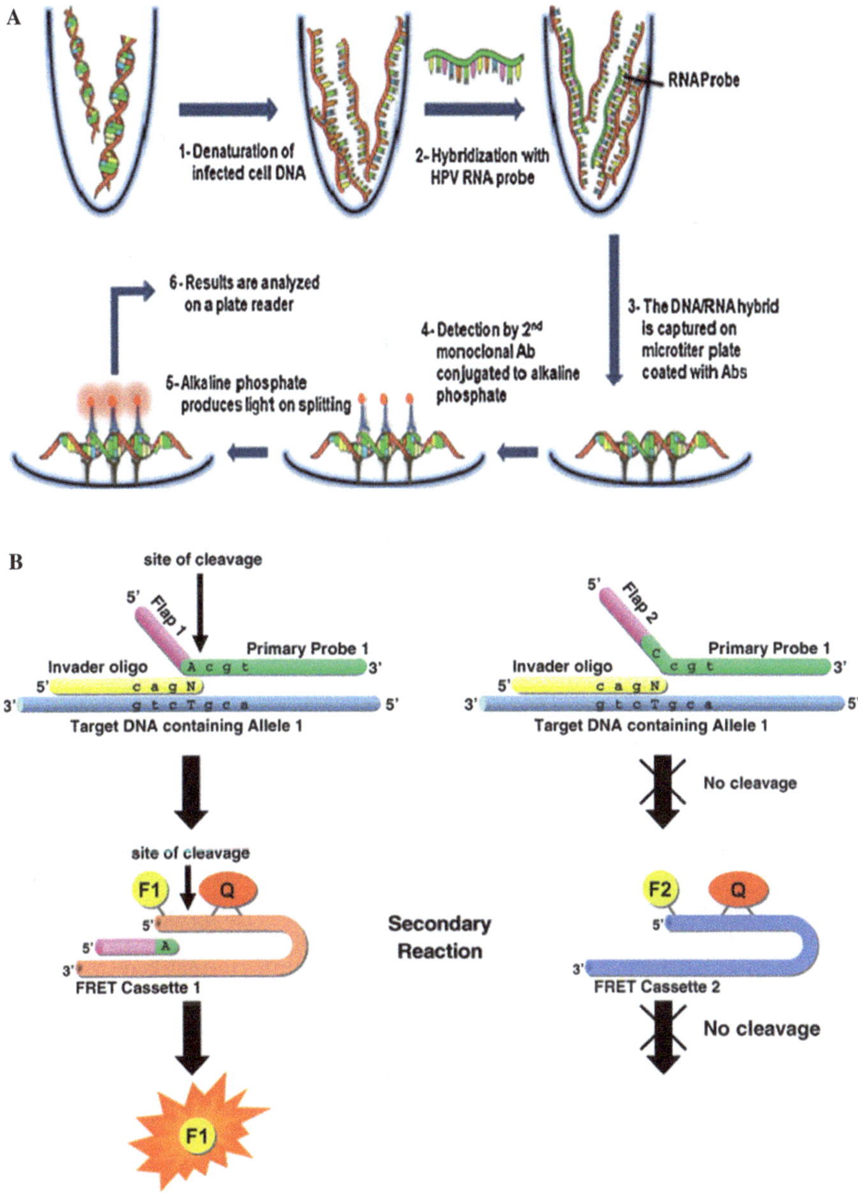

Fig. 4.1 Principle of detection of (**a**) HC2 assay [31], (**b**) Cervista HPV HR assay [32]. (Copyrights Received)

96 well plates coated with the capture antibody are available commercially, having the ability to detect as few as 5000 copies of the viral DNA with a sensitivity of close to 90% [29]. Since 13 hr-HPV probes and 5 lr-HPV probes are simultaneously utilized in

two separate reactions, the assay suffers from cross-reactivity and does not contain an internal control to verify the assay performance, limiting its commercial use [30].

The Cervista HPV HR test is another signal amplification system approved by the FDA in 2009 for HPV detection (14 hr-HPV types) which exploits the isothermal invader DNA assay principle, adopting a Förster resonance energy transfer (FRET)-based readout [33] (Figure 4.1b). The primary phase of the reaction involves the hybridization between the synthetically designed invader oligo and the primary probe with the patient specimen. In the presence of sequence overlap as in Fig. 4.1b, the enzyme cleavase cleaves the probe resulting in a flap. The second phase of the reaction involves the binding of the flap to the universal FRET cassette, resulting in a signal amplification reaction [32]. Unlike the HC2, this assay contains an internal control probe for the human histone 2 gene (H2be), allowing co-analysis with the clinical sample, providing two different coloured readouts and thus ruling out the effect of interferents in sample [34]. While the Cervista HPV HR cannot differentiate between the HPV types, the Cervista HPV 16/18 allows one to determine the presence of either one or both simultaneously [35].

However, the current gold standard technique for the screening of CC is the detection of HPV DNA in the clinical specimens upon PCR amplification. Since close to 98 different genotypes of HPV have been identified and characterized thus far, the primary assay is targeted at amplifying consensus sequences of the HPV L1 gene (not type-specific) using well-established PCR primer sets such as MY09/11 (degenerate primers) [36], GP5+/6+ [37], pGMY09/11 [38] and SPF1/2 (Short PCR fragment) [39]. When more than one genotype of HPV is causing an infection, amplification of consensus sequences results in masking of the genotypes present in a lower concentration and the primers have varied specificities depending on the HPV genotype [40]. Thus, further genotyping is performed using type-specific primers. The GP5+/6+—PCR-EIA is a commercially available assay that primarily utilizes the GP5+/6+ primer pair to amplify a conserved region of the HPV L1 gene and is further coupled with an enzyme immunoassay to further ascertain the genotype of the virus using a set of 13 hr-HPV probes [41].

To perform HPV typing, primers are designed specific to the region of variability between the different HPV genotypes (generally the HPV E6/E7 region). One of the first FDA-approved tests incorporating PCR amplification is the Cobas HPV assay, which is a completely automated assay involving real-time PCR amplification of the HPV L1 gene with a Taqman probe-based readout [42]. Unlike the previously described assays, which are complex in terms of their principle of detection, the Cobas test is rather simple and is divided into four channels with an internal control (β-globin) as in Fig. 4.2a, allowing for genotyping to an extent, since HPV 16, HPV 18 are the most common HPV subtypes causing CC [43].

The Aptima HPV assay is an extension of the amplification-based nucleic acid detection techniques, except that, unlike Cobas, Aptima involve the amplification of RNA instead of DNA [46]. The overall principle of the assay is illustrated in Fig. 4.2c, initially the E6/E7 RNA is captured and further amplified using the technique of transcription-mediated amplification using enzymes such as MMLV reverse transcriptase and T7 polymerase [47]. Further, labelled probes

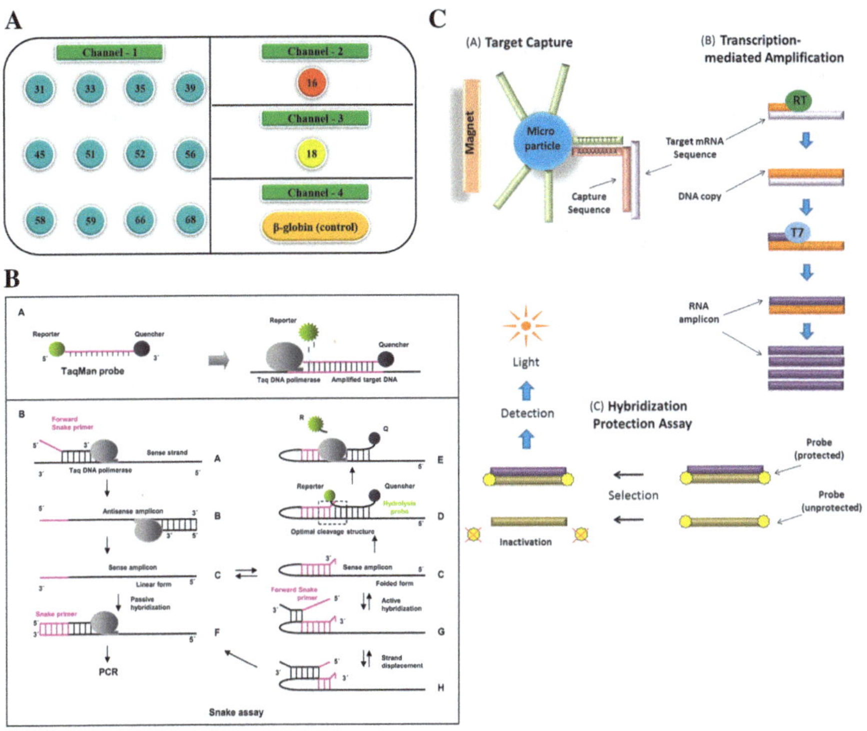

Fig. 4.2 (**a**) Experimental layout of Cobas test, (**b**) Principle of Taq man probe-based qPCR readout [44] (**c**) Principle of detection of Aptima HPV assay [45]. (Copyrights Received)

complementary to the target are introduced in the presence of target, the hybrid is activated by emitting light, while in the absence of the target, no light is emitted as the probes are inactivated. An extension of the assay is the Aptima HPV 16 18/45 genotype assay, which allows for genotyping of the HPV strains in the clinical specimen [48].

4.5 Conclusion

CC screening strategies have evolved over the years at an exponential rate, given the demand for large scale, rapid, sensitive and selective screening tests. In spite of the rapid growth of the industry, for large-scale primary screening of the CC the primitive cytology-based testing (Pap smear test) is being adopted globally, particularly in low resource settings, owing to its affordability and ease of scale up. Slowly, the commercially available HPV tests are replacing Pap smear tests due to their relatively higher sensitivity. Even though a large number of HPV tests have been commercialized, most of the tests either do not perform well analytically or are not well adapted to the real-world point-of-care diagnosis. Thus, automation in the avenues of sample-collection, sample extraction and rapid testing in modular units, establishment of universal standards to test the analytical efficiency of the different tests based on large-scale clinical trials and affordability are aspects of the HPV test kits which need to be improved upon to develop globally usable point-of-care testing systems.

Declaration of Competing Interest The authors declare no conflicts of interest.

Acknowledgements The authors are grateful to the Ministry of Human Resource Development, Government of India for the financial support through *Scheme for Promotion of Academic and Research Collaboration* (*SPARC*) project "SPARC/2018-2019/P402/SL". We also acknowledge the support received from the National Research Foundation (NRF) of Korea for the Basic Science Research Program funded by the Ministry of Education (NRF-2019R1A6A1A03033215). We are grateful to SASTRA Deemed University, India and SKKU, South Korea for providing infrastructural support.

References

1. Tabár L, Gad A, Holmberg LH, Ljungquist U, Fagerberg CJG, Baldetorp L, Gröntoft O, Lundström B, Månson JC, Eklund G et al (1985) Reduction in mortality from breast cancer after mass screening with mammography: randomised trial from the breast cancer screening working Group of the Swedish National Board of health and welfare. Lancet 325:829–832. https://doi.org/10.1016/S0140-6736(85)92204-4
2. Winawer Z et al (1993) Prevention of colorectal cancer by colonscopy polipectomy. N Engl J Med 329(27):1977–1981
3. Soresi M, Magliarisi C, Campagna P, Leto G, Bonfissuto G, Riili A, Carroccio A, Sesti R, Tripi S, Montalto G (2003) Usefulness of alpha-fetoprotein in the diagnosis of hepatocellular carcinoma. Anticancer Res 23:1747–1753
4. Sone S, Li F, Yang ZG, Honda T, Maruyama Y, Takashima S, Hasegawa M, Kawakami S, Kubo K, Haniuda M et al (2001) Results of three-year mass screening programme for lung cancer using mobile low-dose spiral computed tomography scanner. Br J Cancer 84:25–32. https://doi.org/10.1054/bjoc.2000.1531
5. Burd EM (2003) Human papillomavirus and cervical cancer. Clin Microbiol Rev 16:1–17. https://doi.org/10.1128/CMR.16.1.1
6. Storch GA (2000) Diagnostic virology. Clin Infect Dis 31:739–751. https://doi.org/10.1086/314015
7. Ryndock EJ, Biryukov J, Meyers C (2015) Replication of human papillomavirus in culture. Methods Mol Biol 1249:39–52. https://doi.org/10.1007/978-1-4939-2013-6_3
8. Gibson JS (2014) Nucleic acid-based assays for the detection of high-risk human papillomavirus: a technical review. Cancer Cytopathol 122:639–645
9. Michalas SP (2000) The Pap test: George N. Papanicolaou (1883-1962.)A screening test for the prevention of cancer of uterine cervix. Eur J Obstet Gynecol Reprod Biol 90:135–138
10. Raju K (2016) Evolution of Pap stain. Biomed Res Ther 3:490–500. https://doi.org/10.7603/s40730-016-0006-8
11. Klinkhamer PJJM, Meerding WJ, Rosier PFWM, Hanselaar AGJM (2003) Liquid-based cervical cytology. Cancer 99:263–271. https://doi.org/10.1002/cncr.11673
12. Kruse A-J, Baak JPA, Helliesen T, Kjellevold K-H, Robboy SJ (2003) Prognostic value and reproducibility of koilocytosis in cervical intraepithelial neoplasia. Int J Gynecol Pathol Off J Int Soc Gynecol Pathol 22:236–239. https://doi.org/10.1097/01.PGP.0000071045.12278.0A

13. Ancuta E, Sofroni D, Ancuta C, Sofroni L, Mereuta I, Gutu L (2017) Colposcopic assessment among women with lower genital tract pathology. In: Colposcopy and cervical pathology. Intech, London
14. Apgar B, Brotzman G, Spitzer M (2008) Colposcopy - principles and practice, 2nd edn. Saunders, Philadelphia; ISBN 9781437720730
15. Gafirikin L, Lauterbach M, Blumenthal PD (2003) Performance of visual inspection with acetic acid for cervical cancer screening: a qualitative summary of evidence to date. Obstet Gynecol Surv 58:543–550
16. Ghosh P, Gandhi G, Kochhar PK, Zutshi V, Batra S (2012) Visual inspection of cervix with Lugol's iodine for early detection of premalignant & malignant lesions of cervix. Indian J Med Res 136:265–271
17. Oh JK, Shin HR, Gong G, Sohn JH, Khang SK (2008) Diagnostic accuracy of conventional Pap test, liquid-based cytology and human papillomavirus DNA testing in cervical cancer screening in Korea: a meta-analysis. Korean J Epidemiol 30:178–187. https://doi.org/10.4178/kje.2008.30.2.178
18. Di Bonito P, Grasso F, Mochi S, Accardi L, Donà MG, Branca M, Costa S, Mariani L, Agarossi A, Ciotti M et al (2006) Serum antibody response to human papillomavirus (HPV) infections detected by a novel ELISA technique based on denatured recombinant HPV16 L1, L2, E4, E6 and E7 proteins. Infect Agent Cancer 1:1–9. https://doi.org/10.1186/1750-9378-1-6
19. Jeon JH, Shin DM, Cho SY, Song KY, Park NH, Kang HS, Yung DK, Kim IG (2007) Immunocytochemical detection of HPV16 E7 in cervical smear. Exp Mol Med 39:621–628. https://doi.org/10.1038/emm.2007.68
20. Fisher SG, Benitez-Bribiesca L, Nindl I, Stockfleth E, Müller M, Wolf H, Perez-Garcia F, Guzman-Gaona J, Gutierrez-Delgado F, Irvin W et al (1996) The Association of Human Papillomavirus Type 16 E6 and E7 antibodies with stage of cervical cancer. Gynecol Oncol 61:73–78. https://doi.org/10.1006/gyno.1996.0099
21. Rocha-Zavaleta L, Ambrosio JP, de Lourdes Mora-Garcia M, Cruz-Talonia F, Hernandez-Montes J, Weiss-Steider B, Ortiz-Navarrete V, Monroy-Garcia A (2004) Detection of antibodies against a human papillomavirus (HPV) type 16 peptide that differentiate high-risk from low-risk HPV-associated low-grade squamous intraepithelial lesions. J Gen Virol 85:2643–2650. https://doi.org/10.1099/vir.0.80077-0
22. Salazar-Piña DA, Pedroza-Saavedra A, Cruz-Valdez A, Ortiz Panozo E, Maldonado Gama M, Chihu-Amparan L, Rodriguez-Ocampo AN, Orozco-Fararoni E, Esquivel-Guadarrama F, Gutierrez-Xicotencatl L (2016) Validation of serological antibody profiles against human papillomavirus type 16 antigens as markers for early detection of cervical cancer. Medicine (Baltimore) 95:e2769–e2769. https://doi.org/10.1097/MD.0000000000002769
23. Schiffman MH, Bauer HM, Lorincz AT, Manos MM, Byrne JC, Glass AG, Cadell DM, Howley PM (1991) Comparison of southern blot hybridization and polymerase chain reaction methods for the detection of human papillomavirus DNA. J Clin Microbiol 29:573–577. https://doi.org/10.1128/JCM.29.3.573-577.1991
24. Lindh E, Chua KL, Kataoka A, Bistoletti P, Groff D, Hjerpe A (1992) Detection of human papillomavirus (HPV) using dot blot and southern blot, hybridizing with a mixture of seven probes. APMIS 100:301–308. https://doi.org/10.1111/j.1699-0463.1992.tb00876.x
25. Zehbe I, Wilander E, Rylander E, Edlund K, Wadell G (1996) Detection of human papillomavirus in cervical intra-epithelial neoplasia, using in situ hybridization and various polymerase chain reaction techniques. Virchows Arch 428:151–157. https://doi.org/10.1007/BF00200657
26. Coutlée F, Rouleau D, Ferenczy A, Franco E (2005) The laboratory diagnosis of genital human papillomavirus infections. Can J Infect Dis Med Microbiol = J Can des Mal Infect la Microbiol medicale 16:83–91. https://doi.org/10.1155/2005/798710
27. Poljak M, Kocjan BJ, Oštrbenk A, Seme K (2016) Commercially available molecular tests for human papillomaviruses (HPV): 2015 update. J Clin Virol 76:S3–S13. https://doi.org/10.1016/j.jcv.2015.10.023
28. Digene, Hybrid Capture 2 High-Risk HPV DNA Test [Package Insert, 5199–1220]

29. Carozzi FM, Del Mistro A, Confortini M, Sani C, Puliti D, Trevisan R, De Marco L, Tos AG, Girlando S, Palma PD et al (2005) Reproducibility of HPV DNA testing by hybrid capture 2. Am J Clin Pathol 124:716–721. https://doi.org/10.1309/84E5WHJQHK83BGQD
30. Castle PE, Schiffman M, Burk RD, Wacholder S, Hildesheim A, Herrero R, Bratti MC, Sherman ME (2002) Restricted cross-reactivity of hybrid capture 2 with nononcogenic human papillomavirus types. Cancer Epidemiol Biomark Prev 11:1394–1399
31. Ramzan M, Ul Ain N, Ilyas S, Umer M, Bano S, Sarwar S, Shahzad N, Shakoori AR (2015) A cornucopia of screening and diagnostic techniques for human papillomavirus associated cervical carcinomas. J Virol Methods 222:192–201. https://doi.org/10.1016/j.jviromet.2015.06.015
32. Olivier M (2005) The invader® assay for SNP genotyping. Mutat Res Mol Mech Mutagen 573:103–110. https://doi.org/10.1016/j.mrfmmm.2004.08.016
33. Hologic Inc., Cervista HPV HR [Package Insert, PRD-00804, Revision 204]
34. US Food and Drug Administration. Cervista™ HPV HR Labeling. Available online: accessdata.fda.gov/cdrh_docs/pdf8/P080014c.pdf
35. US Food and Drug Administration. Cervista™ HPV 16/18 Labeling. Available online: accessdata.fda.gov/cdrh_docs/pdf8/P080015c.pdf
36. Melchers WJG, Claas HCJ, Quint WGV (1991) Use of the polymerase chain reaction to study the relationship between human papillomavirus infections and cervical cancer. Eur J Clin Microbiol Infect Dis 10:714–727. https://doi.org/10.1007/BF01972496
37. de Roda Husman AM, Walboomers JM, van den Brule AJ, Meijer CJ, Snijders PJ (1995) The use of general primers GP5 and GP6 elongated at their 3′ ends with adjacent highly conserved sequences improves human papillomavirus detection by PCR. J Gen Virol 76(Pt 4):1057–1062. https://doi.org/10.1099/0022-1317-76-4-1057
38. Gravitt PE, Peyton CL, Alessi TQ, Wheeler CM, Coutlée F, Hildesheim A, Schiffman MH, Scott DR, Apple RJ (2000) Improved amplification of genital human papillomaviruses. J Clin Microbiol 38:357–361
39. Kleter B, van Doorn LJ, ter Schegget J, Schrauwen L, van Krimpen K, Burger M, ter Harmsel B, Quint W (1998) Novel short-fragment PCR assay for highly sensitive broad-spectrum detection of anogenital human papillomaviruses. Am J Pathol 153:1731–1739. https://doi.org/10.1016/S0002-9440(10)65688-X
40. Lorincz A, Wheeler CM, Cuschieri K, Geraets D, Meijer CJLM, Quint W (2020) Developing and standardizing human papillomavirus tests; INC; ISBN 9780128144572
41. Snijders PJF, Van Den Brule AJC, Jacobs MV, Pol RP, Meijer CJLM HPV DNA Detection and Typing in Cervical Scrapes. *119*
42. Roche Molecular Systems Inc., Cobas HPV Test [Package Insert, 05641268001, Rev. 1.0]
43. Wright TC, Stoler MH, Behrens CM, Apple R, Derion T, Wright TL (2012) The ATHENA human papillomavirus study: design, methods, and baseline results. Am J Obstet Gynecol 206:46.e1–46.e11. https://doi.org/10.1016/j.ajog.2011.07.024
44. Navarro E, Serrano-Heras G, Castaño MJ, Solera J (2015) Real-time PCR detection chemistry. Clin Chim Acta 439:231–250. https://doi.org/10.1016/j.cca.2014.10.017
45. Bennett KM (2017) In: Coleman WB, Tsongalis GJBT-DMP (eds) Chapter 7 - molecular testing for human papillomaviruses. Academic Press, Cambridge, pp 75–87. ISBN 978-0-12-800886-7
46. Gen-Probe, Aptima HPV Assay [Package Insert, 50218EN, Rev. A]
47. US Food and Drug Administration. APTIMA® HPV Assay Labeling
48. US Food and Drug Administration. APTIMA® HPV 16 18/45 Genotype Assay Labeling. Available online: accessdata.fda.gov/cdrh_docs/pdf12/P120007c

Electrochemical DNA Biosensors for Cervical Cancers

5

Muthaiyan Lakshmanakumar, Noel Nesakumar, Arockia Jayalatha JBB, and John Bosco Balaguru Rayappan

Abstract

Effective diagnosis and preventive approaches can be of great help in reducing the rate of cervical cancer incidence and death. The uses of advanced bio-sensing techniques are crucial in the early diagnosis of cancer, especially for cervical cancer patients that are usually identified at later stages. The development of an affordable clinical diagnostic tool that can be used for the self-testing and clinical analysis of cervical cells is the need of the hour. The electrochemical biosensors were used as important diagnostic technique for cervical cancer analytes and it provides the quantitative/analytical information of the target biomarkers. This chapter highlights the basics, design and development of label-free (direct) and labelled (indirect) DNA-based electrochemical biosensors for the detection of cervical cancer progressed along with the improvements in analytical chemistry. And also, the role of nano-interfaces, challenges in DNA functionalization and

M. Lakshmanakumar · J. B. B. Rayappan (✉)
Centre for Nanotechnology and Advanced Biomaterials (CeNTAB), School of Electrical and Electronics Engineering, SASTRA Deemed University, Thanjavur, Tamil Nadu, India
e-mail: rjbosco@ece.sastra.edu

N. Nesakumar
Centre for Nanotechnology and Advanced Biomaterials (CeNTAB), SASTRA Deemed University, Thanjavur, Tamil Nadu, India

School of Chemical and Biotechnology, SASTRA Deemed University, Thanjavur, Tamil Nadu, India

A. J. JBB
School of Electrical and Electronics Engineering, SASTRA Deemed University, Thanjavur, Tamil Nadu, India

J. B. B. Rayappan, J. H. Lee (eds.), *Biomarkers and Biosensors for Cervical Cancer Diagnosis*, https://doi.org/10.1007/978-981-16-2586-2_5

electrode immobilization have been discussed. Further, the development of point of care (POC) devices with ultrasensitive features for the detection of HPV types 16, 18, and 45 has also been discussed.

Keywords

Electrochemical · Biosensors · DNA · Functionalization · POC

5.1 Introduction

Electrochemical (EC) DNA biosensors have wide benefits such as portability, fast response with better sensitivity, less complexity and are well-suited for mass production using micro-fabrication technology. Most other exceptional detection techniques require costly signal transducer equipment for detecting analytes. Besides, only a few digital instruments might observe very low current signals in the range of pico-amps [1]. EC DNA biosensors are mainly focused on the hybridization of complementary DNA probes or ss-DNA with their target nucleic acid [2]. In recent years, several modern advancements have been accomplished with enhanced interfacial strategies and bio-recognition on solid state devices. With the help of nano-scale accuracy, bio-sensing offers a good diagnosis technique for nucleotide recognition and screening on solid state substrates. Some of the advanced enhancements had been executed recently in this field. The key objective of the DNA biosensor is to aid the formation of a probe target complex, wherein the reaction produces a response, which can be transduced into a detectable signal via EC digital readout.

In EC DNA biosensor, the probe DNA molecules or the ss-DNA are the analytes need to be detected. This simple concept is constructed over the hybridization reaction of the ss-DNA probe towards its complementary DNA. Hybridization causes changes in mass distribution, light absorption or emission characteristic, which will generate the digital output. The output generated is converted into a measurable outcome via an appropriate transduction component including electrochemical, thermal or optical, which transforms the signals into light, current or potential [3].

An EC DNA biosensor popularly works on a three-electrode electrochemical cell, which contains reference, working and counter electrodes [4]. Working electrodes (WE) may include platinum, gold, and carbon electrodes and these electrodes are modified with probe ss-DNA. The platinum wire is employed as a counter electrode and the saturated calomel electrode (SCE) is utilized as a reference electrode. In the EC DNA biosensor, the initial step is to immobilize the DNA probe or ss-DNA on the working electrode surface [5]. The mixture of the ss-DNA probe with the target DNA may initiate reduction/oxidation reactions in the medium and is reflected as changes in the electrochemical signal of the electroactive indicators/labels connected to the probes. The immobilized ss-DNA probe could be bounded on the substrate of WE and detection will be carried out with an EC analyzer. EC biosensors need electroanalytical approaches, including impedometry, conductometry, voltammetry, potentiometric, and amperometry to assess the transduced output signal, which can be employed to describe the electrochemical changes in the system induced by the process of molecular recognition. Owing to their miniature size, rapid response, and low cost, these electrochemical biosensors prove to be a promising diagnostic technique for cervical cancer detection [6].

5.2 Electrochemical Detection of Cervical Cancer

Electrochemical biosensor for the detection of HPV DNA have been a steady increase owing to major benefits such as minimum sample volume requirement, high sensitivity, portability and possibility of large scale manufacturing with the assistance of micro-fabrication devices and point-of-care diagnostics [7]. Every year, the detection of DNA via an electrochemical technique is being carried out and is indicated by increasing publications in this field. However, the limited availability of HPV cervical swab samples is a major bottleneck in validating the efficiency of the newly developed techniques. Electrochemical techniques are classified into direct (label free) and indirect (labelled) methods for the detection of HPV [8].

5.2.1 Label Free Detection of HPV DNA

The direct method (label free) excludes the need for any supporting biomarkers (label), and hence provides simple bio-sensing procedures. Electrochemical DNA biosensors measure the variation of the physiochemical signal on the transducer surface caused by the DNA hybridization shown in Fig. 5.1. Advancement in nanotechnology also improves the electrical transducer signals to detect electrochemical DNA biosensors [9].

Liepold et al. fabricated an innovative numerical microarray design (EDDA) that showed hybridization of DNA within a few minutes. The fabricated dipstick-kind microelectrodes consisted of 32 gold microarray electrodes on a silicon wafer; without any washing procedures or labelling needed, the microelectrodes were directly used for signal amplification reaction. Initially, the probe DNA was functionalized on the gold microelectrodes through the modified DNA-ferrocene hybridization. Immobilization procedures, direct accessibility towards the capture probes and inhibition from non-specific target probes were reported. The target DNA was hybridized to the probe DNA when the fabricated sensor was immersed in the sample. Hence, the electrochemical signal decreased due to the hybridized target DNA. In this direct method, the target DNA (HPV-6) was measured accurately down to the 30 pM range. The sensor also provided reliable and robust performance in scientific laboratories and for diagnosis [10]. Zari et al. immobilized a 20-mer oligonucleotide of HPV on the surface of screen-printed gold electrodes (SPGE) for the detection of hybridized DNA without any redox indicator or label. With the aid of square wave voltammetry (SWV), glassy carbon, gold and carbon paste electrodes are widely used for the detection of DNA probes, adenine, and guanine bases. After acid hydrolysis, SWV was used to determine the guanine and adenine bases. The SPGE showed high sensitivity towards hybridized DNA, the selectivity

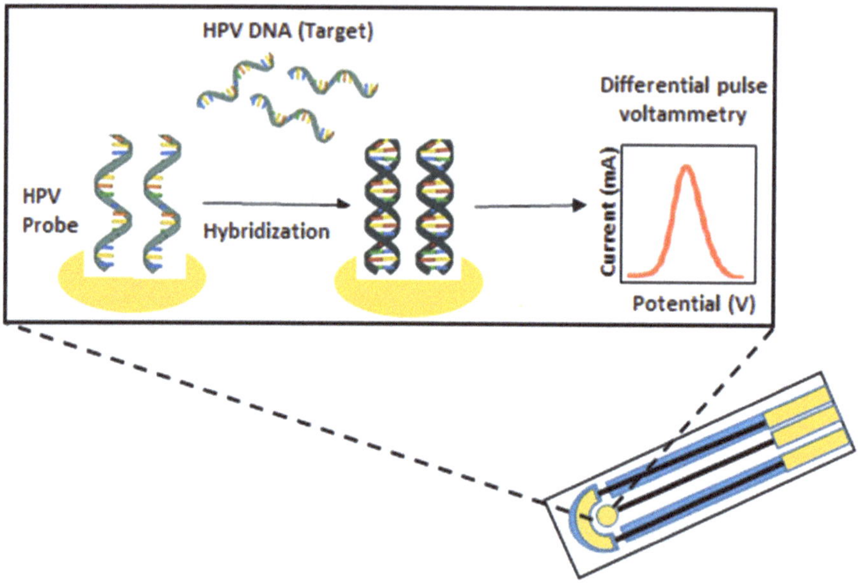

Fig. 5.1 Schematic of electrochemical detection of cervical cancer

of the DNA biosensor was verified with non-complementary oligonucleotide. Also, the HPV DNA sensor displayed a good calibration range with the limit of detection (LOD) of 2 pg/mL. The increase in peak currents was observed to be ordered as follows: probe modified SPGE > 18-base mismatched SPGE > 11-base mismatched modified SPGE > hybrid modified SPGE. The major advantage of this direct method is the suitability of fabricated microarrays and gold screen-printed electrodes to exhibit high sensitivity compared to carbon or mercury electrodes [11]. An immunosensor based on 23-mer oligonucleotide (guanine-free) modified graphite electrode was developed by Campos-Ferreira et al. to recognize E6 gene from HPV 16 virus. The fabricated sensor showed a detection limit of 16 pg/μL. Such a low detection limit enables the fabricated electrode to detect ultra-low concentrations of E6 gene and paves the way for analysis of cloning in plasmid [12].

Piro et al. have built a new technology for the detection of HPV using conjugated copolymer poly (5-hydroxy-1,4-naphthoquinone-co-5-hydroxy-2-carboxyethyl-1,4-naphthoquinone). The immunosensor was proposed to detect HPV-16 (HPV45E6 and HPV16E7p) by using the HPV-16-L1 probe. SWV was used to investigate the anti-HPV(serum), which on interaction produced a strong signal between antigen and antibody [14]. This analytical method also helps to enhance the response of the sensor in terms of stability as well as sensitivity. Dai Tran et al. reported a similar approach using inter-digitated platinum electrode arrays (IDA) modified with polyaniline-multi walled carbon nanotube film (PANi–MWCNT) with a LOD of 490 pM HPV. The sensitivity of the fabricated device is $1.75 \pm 0.2\mu A\ nM^{-1}$ ($R^2 = 0.997$) between 10 and 50 nM of anti-HPV. This study summaries the developed array capability to govern biological and technical deviations.

Furthermore, this work needs to be validated in the real time applications to decide the practicability of the assays [15]. Huang et al. [16] reported label free electrochemical biosensor using glassy carbon electrode (GCE) with graphene/Au nanorod/polythionine (G/Au-NR/PT) and redox indicator of ruthenium complex, $[Ru(phen)^3]^{2+}$ with a LOD of 4.03×10^{-14} M and high selective in the range of 1.0×10^{-13} to 1.0×10^{-10} M [17]. Jampasa et al. [13] have designed and developed a signal-on electrochemical biosensor for the simultaneous detection of HPV type 18 and 16 DNA using a dual-working SPCE electrode shown in Fig. 5.2. They have utilized a signal-on method to improve the signal capacity and dual-working SPCE for the simultaneous detection of type 18 and 16 DNA. Also, they adopted peptide nucleic acid (PNA) rather than DNA with anthraquinone (AQ), a pyrrolidinyl PNA (acpcPNA). The authors have carried out the simultaneous detection of HPV 18 and 16 through sandwich hybridization method. Firstly, the gold nanoparticles were electrodeposited on the SPCE by applying a potential of −0.5 V. The increase in the surface morphology of SPCE due to the deposited Au NPs added advantage by providing more anchoring sites for the PNA capture probes. It is followed by the immobilization of cysteine and an unlabelled capture probe on the gold SPCE electrode in which the amine terminal acts as a cross-linker. The signalling probe, designed to be partially complementary with the 5′ and 3′ positions of the sequence hybridized by the unlabelled probe is covalently attached to the redox species AQ through amide bond formation. It is provisioned with a spacer of 4-base unhybridized gap. The authors have employed differential pulse voltammetry technique for the determination of the DNA target. The oxidation peak at −0.75 V for the AQ labelling agent through sandwich hybridization with the upstream and downstream positions shows a significant difference in the current. A large peak current was observed for HPV 16, while a small peak current is observed for HPV 18. The proposed sensor produced high selectivity without cross-inferences. Further studies have been carried out on the real time samples derived from human cell lines obtained from the PCR technique. The proposed sensor produced a linear response over the range of 0.5–100 nM and a LOQ of 0.5 nM for both DNA strains and a LOD of 153 and 150 pM for type 18 and 16, respectively. The choice of amplification reaction is important in the homogeneous bio-sensing strategy without labelling for the detection of HPV16 E7 and E6 oncogenes [18]. They have adopted hyperbranched rolling circle amplification (HRCA) technique solely driven by the entropy of the system. The diffusivity of the electrochemical indicator is responsible for the resulting electrochemical signal. In the absence of the target DNA the amplification process will not take place and most of the methylene blue (MB) shows a high diffusion coefficient to the electrode. In the presence of target DNA, it facilitates the entropy-driven target recycling process. The target DNA binds with the triple-stranded complex and results in the strand displacement reaction in-turn it can catalyse the entropy-driven amplification reaction. Further, the hybridization generates circular padlock probes. The HRCA helps in the production of a large number of ss-DNA and ds-DNA. The resultant fragments can easily embed the methylene blue indicator. The strong electrostatic repulsion between the negative charged ITO working electrode and the DNA restricts the diffusion of MB over the electrode surface, which results in a reduced electrochemical signal. The

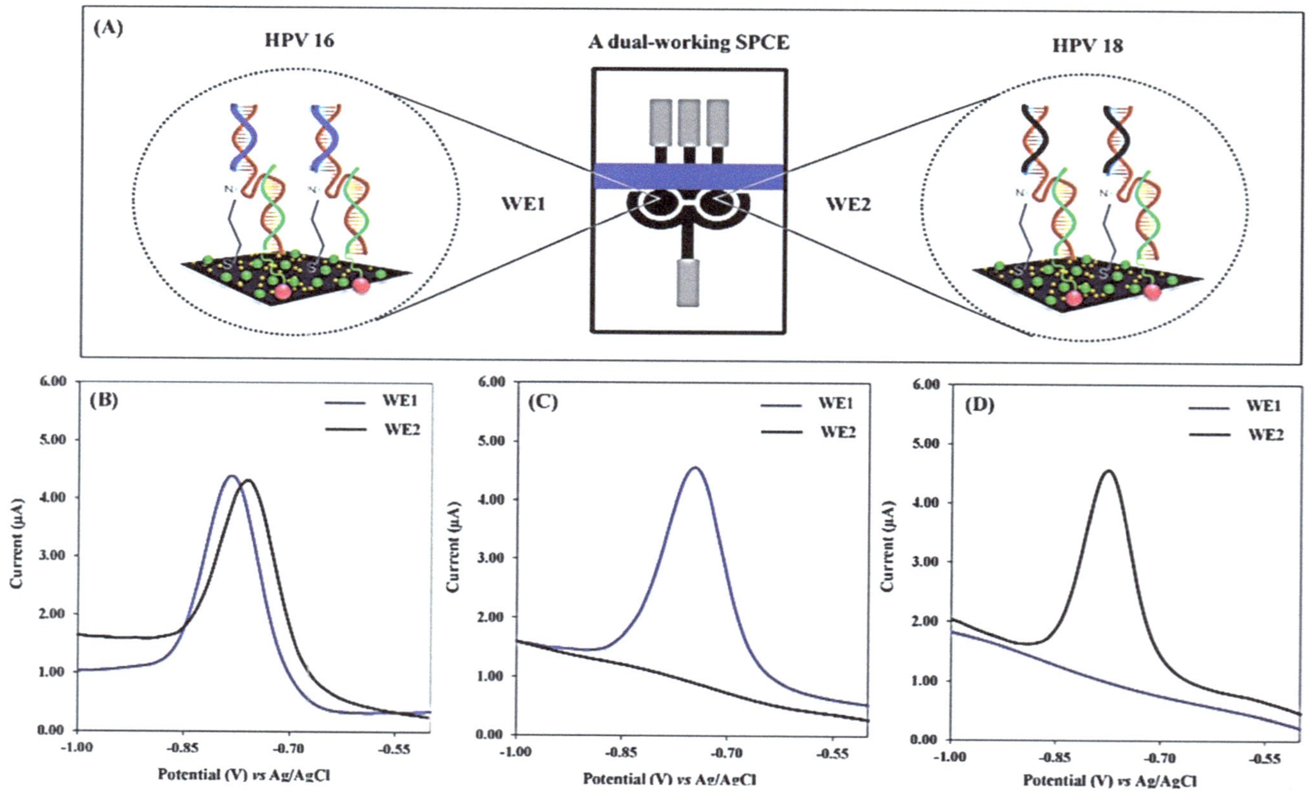

Fig. 5.2 Schematic illustration of a dual-working electrode where a specific probe was immobilized (**a**). DPVs response for the simultaneous detection of HPV type 16 and 18 DNA (**b**). Cross-interference assay of the proposed sensor for type 16 (**c**) and 18 (**d**) at 100 nM DNA concentration in PBS pH 7.4 [13]. (Copyright Received)

target concentration is directly related to the electrochemical signal, which is observed using the differential pulse voltammetry (DPV) technique in the range of −0.1 to −0.6 V. The authors have also carried out agarose gel electrophoresis and fluorescence measurement for the confirmation of the signal amplification. Wherein no bands were found in the g, h, and i lane which strongly routes for the proposed entropy-driven amplification reaction of the target DNA. The authors have optimized the embedded time and concentration to be 60 min and 40μM. The designed sensor produces a linear response and a low detection limit of 0.1 fM to 10 pM and 18.6 attomole, respectively. Further, the authors have done studies on clinical samples obtained from cervical patients. Karimizefreh et al. [19] have improved electrochemical detection of HPV by modifying the GCE with gold nanosheet, as the active sites on gold nanosheet, such as edges and corners, played a major role to increase its sensitivity [16]. The thiolated single-stranded 25-mer oligonucleotide (synthetic thiol-ss-DNA) was immobilized on gold nanosheet and the LOD was found to be 0.15 pM. Regarding the electrochemical DNA biosensor for sensing HPV 16 in human blood serum samples, the authors have developed a new portable PCR free method for detection of HPV 16 [12]. They have fabricated a highly sensitive electrochemical DNA biosensor for the recognition of HPV 16. Primarily they prepared a cysteine film through electrodeposition by applying a potential in the range of −0.2 to 1.5 V. Further, the HPV-16 specific probe was immobilized by adsorption over the film. Due to its special functionalities, this particular amino acid has been adopted as bridge between the working electrode and the HPV 16 probe through ionic interactions. The authors have utilized the DPV technique to monitor the hybridization of the specific probe with synthetic targets as well as from clinical samples. They performed the studies using MB as a redox reporter for pre- and post-hybridization processes. The effect of hybridization results in a significant decrease in the MB signal. The reduction of MB was carried out between −0.6 and 0 V. The authors have optimized the probe concentration to be 1000 nM with a high current signal. The low concentration produces low current signal due to the less availability of surface probes and high concentration leads to probe overlapping, which results in less number of guanine bases followed by less reduction of MB. The authors have further carried out the work with DNA extracts from cervical swabs of HPV positive patients. Also, they performed a confirmation study on the clinical samples using PCR technique. The proposed sensor produced a linear response in the range of 18.75 nM and 250 nM and a detection limit of 18.13 nM.

PEGylation promotes protein-PEG complex formation, preserves biological activity at neutral pH and is widely used for biological applications. In this regard, Chandra et al. [20] utilized PEGylated-arginine (PA) towards impedimetric detection of cervical cancer HeLa cells. Viscous solution of PEGylated-arginine obtained from vacuum evaporation of the reaction mixture formulated using di(ethyleneglycol)-ethyl ether acrylate and dried methanolic suspension. The prepared PA was purified and used for stabilising Fe_3O_4 magnetic nanoparticles (MNP) synthesised via a co-precipitation method. GCEs were modified with the prepared PA-MNPs incubated in Immunoglobulin G (IgG) solution for 6 h. Following this, the response of electrodes towards different cell lines such as breast cancer cell lines and normal mouse fibroblast cell lines were studied. In similar lines, the inoculated HeLa cells bound to the IgG/PA-MNP modified electrode were allowed to grow. Following this, for varying concentrations of drugs, doxorubicin, methotrexate, and hydroxyurea, the effects on cell viability were studied. Towards this, the peak current at 0.3 V, which corresponds to reduction of disulfide bonds (in HeLa cells) decreased on addition of doxorubicin was observed. On the other hand, a dip in peak current at 0.2 V corresponding to reduction of amino groups on addition of methotrexate was observed. Further, confocal microscopy imaging revealed sufficient cell internalization of drugs and MNPs. Electrochemical Impedance Spectroscopy (EIS) measurements were in direct correlation, with charge transfer resistance (Rct) increasing linearly with the logarithm of the concentration of cells attached to the electrode surface. The sensor exhibited appreciable SNR characteristics and the LOD was reported to be 10 cells mL^{-1} [20].

5.2.2 Labelled (Indirect) Detection of DNA

Even though the label free detection of HPV DNA requires simple screening procedures and reduces the time consumption and cost, the sensitivity level of label free technique is lesser compared to the labelled DNA detection technique. The labelled (indirect) electrochemical technique can detect DNA concentrations down to attomole. The labelled technique requires mediators, such as MB Fe $[(CN)]_6^{3-/4-}$, $[Ru(bpy)3]^{3+/2+}$, ferrocene and $Os(bpy)^3$, which enhances the electron transfer between the DNA and electrode. The indirect electrochemical method could also utilize metal nanoparticles, which also play a significant role as redox mediators to detect the target DNA [5].

Sabzi et al. have designed a renewable transducer pencil graphite electrode (PGE) designed for the detection of HPV target DNA [8]. They have utilized oligonucleotide as a DNA probe and MB as an electroactive reporter. The hybridization of the probe and its complementary DNA is monitored by the MB signal. The activation of the prepared transducer is carried out by tracking the MB signals, in conditions where 1.5 V and 450 s are fixed as the optimum potential and time, respectively. Secondly, the probe immobilization plays a crucial role in the performance of the sensor. The immobilization at the negative potential helps in the MB accumulation. The authors have utilized square wave voltammetry to understand the hybridization reaction. The MB signals decreased substantially in the presence of complementary DNA. The sensor provided great selectivity towards HPV DNA and the detection limit of 1.2 $ng\mu l^{-1}$.

Nasirzadeh et al. used hematoxylin as an electroactive indicator for the detection of HPV DNA [19]. The detection is governed by the interaction between hematoxylin and the target analyte. The authors have done an optimization study for the probe and the hybridization of the target analytes. Here, the authors have investigated two types of immobilization strategies such as droplet and solution self-assembly. Hence, the droplet technique provides a high accumulation signal. Also, a large signal was obtained after the hybridization process. The authors have carried out a comparison study for different hybridization techniques such as drop, preheated solution, and solution hybridization method. Among all, the solution hybridization method gives comparatively better results because the target DNA can choose the most suitable orientation and the optimum time for the hybridization process. The authors used differential pulse voltammetry and cyclic voltammetry for the detection of HPV DNA. The voltammetry signals clearly distinguish the complementary, non-complementary, and the mismatch DNA sequence. The current response for the hematoxylin increases initially till 8.0μM and it then decreases with increasing probe concentration due to the unavailability of interaction site between the electroactive indicator and the target DNA. They observed an increase of hematoxylin signal with ds-DNA in comparison to the ss-DNA. The proposed sensor produced a linear response at the concentration range of 12.5–350.0 nM and a LOD of 3.8 nM. Jampasa et al. have designed the labelled anthraquinone-pyrrolidinyl peptide nucleic acid (acpcPNA) probe for HPV 16 sensing. The SPCE/chitosan is immobilized with an acpcPNA probe linked through a C-terminal lysine residue glutaraldehyde as mediator. Linear detection range between 0.02 and 12.0μM, limit of quantification and LOD of 14 and 4 nM were observed [21]. This fabricated electrode appears to have high selectivity and has the ability to be used effectively in PCR tests to identify HPV 16 DNA. The sensor is economical to manufacture and needs only a limited sample volume. The bio-sensing device is indeed easy and this analytical technique can be used as an innovative screening approach for effective HPV monitoring in developing countries. The limitations of this method involve the need to immobilize the PNA probe, the lack of regeneration and the very high detection limit provided by the DNA detection method. Yet, the limit of detection is reasonably better to enable HPV type 16 DNA to be detected from PCR samples. Civit et al. have fabricated a genosensor array developed for the detection of three HPV DNA [22]. Primarily, the mixture of thiolated probes and bipodal alkanethiol have been immobilized on a 4 × 4 array electrode through co-immobilization. They used a sandwich type hybridization technique for the simultaneous detection of HPV types 16, 18, and 45. This multiplexed array helps in the screening of multiple analytes. The three probes for the three HPV types were immobilized alternatively among the 16 gold working electrodes. The target detection takes place through the hybridization of the specific HRP-labelled probe. The authors have also verified the genotype sensor with the amplified clinical samples. The designed sensor produces high specificity for the target analytes with a low background signal for the non-specific analytes with high reproducibility. The sensor produces a LOD of about 220 pM, 170 pM, and 110 pM, for HPV type 16, 18, and 45, respectively. The quantitative analysis of clinical samples was carried out and the sensor was able to produce a high degree of correlation with the laboratory analysis. The adapted platform could be widely employed as it has the ability to multiplex and can detect nucleic acids with greater precision, especially in identifying RNA expression profiles in theranostics. The electrochemical sensors have a huge linear range and low LOD, in comparison to other DNA biosensors depicted in Table 5.1. In the cutting-edge world, the development of high-quality biosensor for cervical cancer prevention could be possible.

Table 5.1 Comparison of electrochemical biosensor for HPV Detection [23]. (Copyright Received)

Electrochemical technique	Electrode	Electroactive label	Detection limit	Linear range	Reference
DPV	L-cysteine film/gold electrode	Methylene blue	18.13 nM	18.75–250 nM	[12]
	Graphene/Au nanorod /polythionine/GCE	([Ru(phen)^3]$^{2+}$)	4.03 × 10^{-5} M	10^{-4}–10^{-1} nM	[17]
	Pencil graphite electrode	Label free	16 pg/μL	40–5000 pg/μL	[24]
	Graphite electrode	Methylene blue	1.49 nM	2–10 nM	[25]
CV and DPV	Gold electrode	Hematoxylin	3.8 nM	12.5–350 nM	[19]
Steps and sweeps	Oligonucleotide/Gold electrodes	Horseradish peroxidase	490 pM	0.1–10 nM	[7]
Steps and sweeps	Gold electrodes	Horseradish peroxidase	220 pM	0.1–10 nM	[26]
SWV	Pencil graphite electrode	Methylene blue	1.2 ng/μL	0–10 ng/μL	[8]
SWV	Carboxyphenyl layer/GCE	Mercury(II)	$1.2 \cdot 10^{-5}$	10^{-15}–10^{-6} M	[9]
SWV	Screen-printed gold electrode	Label free	2 pg ml^{-1}	0–5 ng ml^{-1}	[11]
SWV	Poly(HNQ-co-HNQ-COOH) film/GCE	Label free	50 nM	–	[14]
CV and SWV	Inter-digitated platinum electrode array/polyaniline/multi-walled carbon nanotube film	Label free	490 pM	10–50 nM	[15]
SWV	Screen-printed carbon/chitosan	Anthraquinone	4.0 nM	.02–12μM	[27]
EIS & SWV	Graphene/Polyaniline	Pyrrolidinyl	2.3 nM	10–200 nM	[28]
ACV&CV	Dipstick-type microelectrode gold arrays	Ferrocenium	30 pM	–	[10]
Amperometry	Glassy carbon/ carbon nano-onion	Horseradish peroxidase	0.54 nM	0–20 nM	[29]
EIS	Single walled carbon nanotube arrays/Au nanoparticles/SiO_2/Si substrate	Label free	10^{-9} M	10^{-9} - 10^{-3} nM	[30]

5.3 Conclusion

The design and development of effective biosensors for the detection of cervical cancer in underdeveloped countries remains a major obstacle. Clinical diagnostics requires significant advancements and is primarily focused on the emergence of novel materials for the construction of rapid and sensitive biosensors. The development of an affordable clinical diagnostic tool that can be used for the self-testing and clinical analysis of cervical cells is the need of the hour, and the deployment of these analytical tools allows detection of cervical cells in patients residing in middle- and low-income countries. Another downside of existing detection techniques is the lack of personal testing, owing to the need for chemical reagents and sample pre-treatment. Therefore, HPV biosensors need new technological improvements with an effective sensing platform capable of detecting and quantifying ultra-low concentrations of HPV in cervical cells without compromising accuracy and precision.

Declaration of Competing Interest The authors declare no conflicts of interest.

Acknowledgements Authors are grateful to the Ministry of Human Resource Development, Government of India for the financial support through *Scheme for Promotion of Academic and Research Collaboration* (*SPARC*) project "SPARC/2018-2019/P402/SL". We also acknowledge the support received from the National Research Foundation (NRF) of Korea for the Basic Science Research Program funded by the Ministry of Education (NRF-2019R1A6A1A03033215). We are grateful to SASTRA Deemed University, India and SKKU, South Korea for providing infrastructural support.

References

1. Drummond TG, Hill MG, Barton JK (2003) Electrochemical DNA sensors. Nat Biotechnol 21:1192–1199
2. Tosar JP, Branas G, Laiz J (2010) Electrochemical DNA hybridization sensors applied to real and complex biological samples. Biosens Bioelectron 26:1205–1217
3. Sassolas A, Leca-Bouvier BD, Blum LJ (2008) DNA biosensors and microarrays. Chem Rev 108:109–139
4. Ronkainen NJ, Halsall HB, Heineman WR (2010) Electrochemical biosensors. Chem Soc Rev 39:1747–1763
5. Ozkan D, Kara P, Kerman K, Meric B, Erdem A, Jelen F, Nielsen PE, Ozsoz M (2002) DNA and PNA sensing on mercury and carbon electrodes by using methylene blue as an electrochemical label. Bioelectrochemistry 58:119–126
6. Teles FRR, Fonseca LP (2008) Trends in DNA Biosensors. Talanta 77:606–623
7. Civit L, Fragoso A, O'Sullivan CK (2010) Electrochemical biosensor for the multiplexed detection of human papillomavirus genes. Biosens Bioelectron 26:1684–1687. https://doi.org/10.1016/j.bios.2010.06.072
8. Sabzi RE, Sehatnia B, Pournaghi-Azar MH, Hejazi MS (2008) Electrochemical detection of human papilloma virus (HPV) target DNA using MB on pencil graphite electrode. J Iran Chem Soc 5:476–483. https://doi.org/10.1007/BF03246005
9. Wang J, Jiang M, Mukherjee B (1999) Flow detection of nucleic acids at a conducting polymer-modified electrode. Anal Chem 71:4095–4099

10. Liepold P, Kratzmüller T, Persike N, Bandilla M, Hinz M, Wieder H, Hillebrandt H, Ferrer E, Hartwich G (2008) Electrically detected displacement assay (EDDA): a practical approach to nucleic acid testing in clinical or medical diagnosis. Anal Bioanal Chem 391:1759–1772. https://doi.org/10.1007/s00216-008-2045-5
11. Zari N, Amine A, Ennaji MM (2009) Label-free DNA biosensor for electrochemical detection of short DNA sequences related to human papilloma virus. Anal Lett 42:519–535. https://doi.org/10.1080/00032710802421897
12. Campos-Ferreira DS, Nascimento GA, Souza EVM, Souto-Maior MA, Arruda MS, Zanforlin DML, Ekert MHF, Bruneska D, Lima-Filho JL (2013) Electrochemical DNA biosensor for human papillomavirus 16 detection in real samples. Anal Chim Acta 804:258–263. https://doi.org/10.1016/j.aca.2013.10.038
13. Jampasa S, Siangproh W, Laocharoensuk R, Yanatatsaneejit P, Vilaivan T, Chailapakul O (2018) A new DNA sensor design for the simultaneous detection of HPV type 16 and 18 DNA. Sensors Actuators B Chem 265:514–521. https://doi.org/10.1016/j.snb.2018.03.045
14. Piro B, Kapella A, Le VH, Anquetin G, Zhang QD, Reisberg S, Noel V, Tran LD, Duc HT, Pham MC (2011) Towards the detection of human papillomavirus infection by a reagentless electrochemical peptide biosensor. Electrochim Acta 56:10688–10693. https://doi.org/10.1016/j.electacta.2011.04.094
15. Tran LD, Nguyen DT, Nguyen BH, Do QP, Le Nguyen H (2011) Development of interdigitated arrays coated with functional polyaniline/MWCNT for electrochemical biodetection: application for human papilloma virus. Talanta 85:1560–1565. https://doi.org/10.1016/j.talanta.2011.06.048
16. Karimizefreh A, Mahyari FA, VaezJalali M, Mohammadpour R, Sasanpour P (2017) Impedimetic biosensor for the DNA of the human papilloma virus based on the use of gold nanosheets. Microchim Acta 184:1729–1737. https://doi.org/10.1007/s00604-017-2173-8
17. Huang H, Bai W, Dong C, Guo R, Liu Z (2015) An ultrasensitive electrochemical DNA biosensor based on graphene/Au Nanorod/Polythionine for human papillomavirus DNA detection. Biosens Bioelectron 68:442–446
18. He Y, Cheng L, Yang Y, Chen P, Qiu B, Guo L, Wang Y, Lin Z, Hong G (2020) Label-free homogeneous electrochemical biosensor for HPV DNA based on entropy-driven target recycling and Hyperbranched rolling circle amplification. Sensors Actuators B Chem 320:128407. https://doi.org/10.1016/j.snb.2020.128407
19. Nasirizadeh N, Zare HR, Pournaghi-Azar MH, Hejazi MS (2011) Introduction of Hematoxylin as an electroactive label for DNA biosensors and its employment in detection of target DNA sequence and Single-Base mismatch in human papilloma virus corresponding to oligonucleotide. Biosens Bioelectron 26:2638–2644. https://doi.org/10.1016/j.bios.2010.11.026
20. Chandra S, Barola N, Bahadur D (2011) Impedimetric biosensor for early detection of cervical cancer. Chem Commun 47:11258–11260. https://doi.org/10.1039/c1cc14547a
21. Jampasa S, Wonsawat W, Rodthongkum N, Siangproh W, Yanatatsaneejit P, Vilaivan T, Chailapakul O (2014) Electrochemical detection of human papillomavirus DNA type 16 using a Pyrrolidinyl peptide nucleic acid probe immobilized on screen-printed carbon electrodes. Biosens Bioelectron 54:428–434. https://doi.org/10.1016/j.bios.2013.11.023
22. Civit L, Fragoso A, Hölters S, Dürst M, O'Sullivan CK (2012) Electrochemical genosensor array for the simultaneous detection of multiple high-risk human papillomavirus sequences in clinical samples. Anal Chim Acta 715:93–98
23. Rasouli E, Shahnavaz Z, Basirun WJ, Rezayi M, Avan A, Ghayour-Mobarhan M, Khandanlou R, Johan MR (2018) Advancements in electrochemical DNA sensor for detection of human papilloma virus - a review. Anal Biochem 556:136–144. https://doi.org/10.1016/j.ab.2018.07.002
24. Campos-Ferreira DS, Souza EVM, Nascimento GA, Zanforlin DML, Arruda MS, Beltrão MFS, Melo AL, Bruneska D, Lima-Filho JL (2016) Electrochemical DNA biosensor for the detection of human papillomavirus E6 gene inserted in recombinant plasmid. Arab J Chem 9:443–450. https://doi.org/10.1016/j.arabjc.2014.05.023

25. Souza E, Nascimento G, Santana N, Campos-ferreira D, Bibiano J, Arruda MS (2014) Electrochemical DNA biosensor for sequences related to the human papillomavirus type 16 using methylene blue. Biosens J 3:3–7
26. Civit L, Fragoso A, Hölters S, Dürst M, O'Sullivan CK (2012) Electrochemical genosensor array for the simultaneous detection of multiple high-risk human papillomavirus sequences in clinical samples. Anal Chim Acta 715:93–98. https://doi.org/10.1016/j.aca.2011.12.009
27. Jampasa S, Wonsawat W, Rodthongkum N, Siangproh W, Yanatatsaneejit P, Vilaivan T, Chailapakul O (2014) Electrochemical detection of human papillomavirus DNA type 16 using a Pyrrolidinyl peptide nucleic acid probe immobilized on screen-printed carbon electrodes. Biosens Bioelectron 54:428–434
28. Teengam P, Siangproh W, Tuantranont A, Henry CS, Vilaivan T, Chailapakul O (2017) Electrochemical paper-based peptide nucleic acid biosensor for detecting human papillomavirus. Anal Chim Acta 952:32–40. https://doi.org/10.1016/j.aca.2016.11.071
29. Bartolome JP, Echegoyen L, Fragoso A (2015) Reactive carbon Nano-onion modified glassy carbon surfaces as DNA sensors for human papillomavirus oncogene detection with enhanced sensitivity. Anal Chem 87:6744–6751
30. Wang S, Li L, Jin H, Yang T, Bao W, Huang S, Wang J (2013) Electrochemical detection of hepatitis B and papilloma virus DNAs using SWCNT array coated with gold nanoparticles. Biosens Bioelectron 41:205–210

Optical DNA Based Sensors for Cervical Cancers

6

Jun Hyuk Heo, Jin Woong Lee, Shrute Kannappan, and
Jung Heon Lee

Abstract

Optical biosensors are devices frequently used to detect different molecules in biological applications through their interaction with light. Optical biosensors have many advantages because they allow fast and direct detection of target molecules. So, they can be easily applied to different types of delicate or miniature point-of-care devices with high reliability. Although many different types of optical platforms are used in biosensing, fluorescent and colorimetric sensors have mostly been adapted for the detection of cervical cancer. Many studies are reporting rapid, low-cost, and disposable biosensors using fluorescently labeled

J. H. Heo · J. W. Lee
School of Advanced Materials Science and Engineering, Sungkyunkwan University (SKKU), Suwon, South Korea

Research Center for Advanced Materials Technology, Sungkyunkwan University (SKKU), Suwon, South Korea

S. Kannappan
Research Center for Advanced Materials Technology, Sungkyunkwan University (SKKU), Suwon, South Korea

Department of Molecular Cell Biology, School of Medicine, Sungkyunkwan University (SKKU), Suwon, South Korea

J. H. Lee (✉)
School of Advanced Materials Science and Engineering, Research Center for Advanced Materials Technology, Biomedical Institute for Convergence at SKKU (BICS), Sungkyunkwan University (SKKU), Suwon, Republic of Korea
e-mail: jhlee7@skku.edu

J. B. B. Rayappan, J. H. Lee (eds.), *Biomarkers and Biosensors for Cervical Cancer Diagnosis*, https://doi.org/10.1007/978-981-16-2586-2_6

probes with various fluorophores to detect human papillomavirus (HPV) DNA in a single assay. However, fluorescent biosensors can be adapted with nanoparticles, microbeads, and two-dimensional nanomaterials, and even Clustered regularly interspaced short palindromic repeats—CRISPR associated (CRISPR-Cas) for an improved limit of detection, easy separation of probes, simplification of sensor design and operation, etc. Similarly, many colorimetric sensors have been reported for the detection of different types of HPV DNA. Colorimetric sensors have a unique advantage as detection can be carried out with naked eyes without the need for any instrument but only has relatively moderate sensitivity. Additional techniques, such as loop-mediated isothermal amplification, DNAzymes, peptide nucleic acid, can be incorporated to improve its detection limit significantly. Besides, both fluorescence and colorimetric sensors can be applied to lateral flow assays, microfluidic systems, or microarrays for rapid and multiplexed detection of HPV. In this chapter, recent progress in the DNA-based optical biosensors for cervical cancer detection is summarized with emphasis on fluorescent and colorimetric sensors.

Keywords

Optical biosensor · Fluorescence · Colorimetric · DNA · Cervical cancer · HPV

6.1 Introduction

Optical biosensors are a class of devices used to detect different molecules in biological applications through their interaction with light [1–5]. They consist of a light source that generates electromagnetic waves, a biosensing platform where the light and molecules interact, and a detector that distinguishes and assesses electromagnetic wave spectrum as they interact with target molecules [6–8]. The principle of an optical biosensor is premised on the variation in the typical signals from an optical platform, which is caused by specific biological interactions occurring in the presence of target molecules [9, 10].

Design and engineering of an optical biosensor are important to significantly increase its sensitivity and selectivity and make it suitable for practical use. Recently, nanotechnology opened up a new path to develop highly advanced biosensing platforms with excellent optical properties [11–13]. These nano-platforms could be correlated with different spectroscopic methods including fluorescence, surface enhanced Raman spectroscopy (SERS), localized surface plasmon resonance (LSPR), and surface plasmon resonance (SPR), which can be developed into the form of the newest biosensing system [9, 10, 14–18]. Especially, optical biosensors have many advantages because they allow fast and direct detection of target molecules. So, they can be easily adapted into different types of delicate or miniature point of care (POC) devices with high reliability. Although many different types of optical biosensors exist, fluorescent and colorimetric sensors have been adapted for the detection of HPV.

One of the earliest methods adopted for the detection of HPV includes FISH (Fluorescent in situ hybridization) which involves the treatment of tissue samples with fluorescently labeled DNA probes to identify the presence of HPV DNA. This method, however, is laborious, time-taking, and is rather a qualitative assay [19]. Thus, with the advent of DNA amplification strategies such as polymerase chain reaction (PCR), quantitative detection of HPV DNA using fluorescent probes is now possible and is being widely studied in the last few decades.

6.2 Fluorescent Biosensors

Fluorescence-based detection technique has been widely developed as an essential analytical tool in drug discovery and disease identification [20, 21]. This technique has been actively used to recognize HPV specific genotype such as HPV-45, HPV-16, and HPV-18 in a quantitative manner [22]. It is well known that fluorescently labeled probes with various fluorophores can be used for rapid, low cost, and disposable biosensors in a single assay to detect HPV DNA [23, 24]. A recent study by Wang et al. reports a sandwich assay for simultaneous detection of HPV-18 and HPV-16 using silica nanoparticles (NPs). In this assay, one-step hybridization reaction can happen simply by mixing biotinylated capture DNA modified NPs, target DNAs (HPV-18 and HPV-16), and 6-carboxyl-X-rhodamine (Rox) or fluorescein amidite (FAM) labeled HPV-18 and HPV-16 probes. Subsequently, centrifugation isolated the hybrid-conjugated NPs, and finally, the fluorescence signals of Rox and FAM were identified (Fig. 6.1a). The limits of detection (LOD) for HPV-16 and HPV-18 were 0.17 nM and 0.78 nM, respectively [25]. Instead of conjugating the fluorophore to the DNA probe as in the previously discussed study, Riccò et al. have directly entrapped the fluorophore (Alexa Fluor® 555) within the streptavidin modified silica NP through biotin-streptavidin interaction and further attached amine-modified DNA probes onto the NPs. The luminescent NPs thus obtained were applied to a microarray system to detect various high-risk HPV types. The platform developed, despite the technical difficulties in terms of synthesis, was found to have a better signal intensity than commercial QDs (12 times higher) with a detection limit of 20 pM [26].

Besides, there are some studies reporting the detection of HPV DNA strands using quantum dots (QDs) modified with various kinds of fluorophore-labeled random DNA, which were used as labels for the detection of HPV DNA strands, including HPV-45, HPV-18, and HPV-16. Magnetic microparticles (MMPs) or nanoparticles (MNPs) were also utilized for separation of samples after hybridization. Consequentially, certain HPV could be clearly identified simply by measuring the fluorophore signals [28, 29]. In addition to paramagnetic QDs, non-magnetic CdTe QDs have been utilized by Shamsipur et al. for the detection of HPV-18 via fluorescence resonance energy transfer (FRET). In the absence of the target, the Cy5 labeled probe and the QD modified with the probe are far apart, effectively emitting fluorescence. However, in the presence of the HPV target, hybridization with the probe occurs and thence Cy5 and QD are in proximity. So

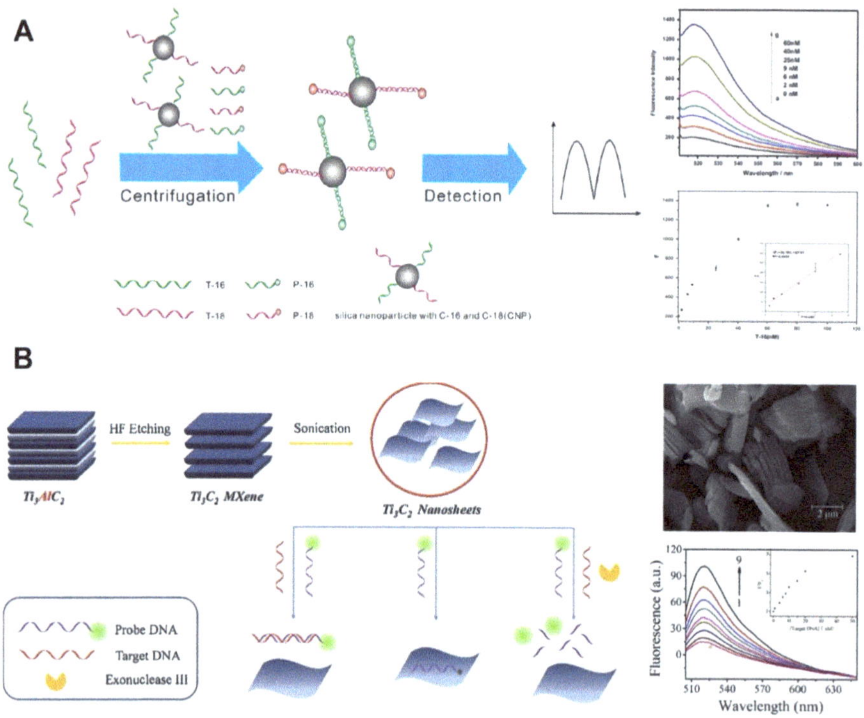

Fig. 6.1 (**a**) Schematic of multiplex detection of HPV DNAs (HPV-16 and HPV-18) using silica nanoparticles (NPs) functionalized with capture probes as the sensing platform [25]. (**b**) Schematic of the analysis of HPV-18 DNA using MXene as a 2D sensing material [27]. (Copyrights Received)

Cy5 acts as an acceptor and yields a linear variation in fluorescence intensity in a concentration-dependent manner (1–50 nM) [30].

Recently, two-dimensional (2D) nanosheets such as graphene (GO), MXenes, and transition metal dichalcogenides (TMDCs) were regarded as promising materials with ultrahigh quenching efficiencies of fluorophores, due to the nanoscale-surface energy transfer (NSET) [31–34]. Zhang et al. suggested a homogenous assay platform for the detection of HPV DNA using polyethylene glycol (PEG)-PtS_2 nanosheet combined with fluorophores. This method has advantages because it is possible to detect HPV DNA without the need of probe immobilization and washing steps [35]. Also, it has been reported that Ti_3C_2 MXene has a high fluorescence quenching efficiency of fluorophores and the detection of HPV-18 can be performed in a "off-on" type manner (Fig. 6.1b) [27].

In another studies, a microfluidic device containing microbead array was suggested to identify or quantify the HPV DNA such as HPV-16 and HPV-18 [36, 37]. Microbeads were used to capture probes for the detection of HPV DNA in a microfluidic channel. Through "sandwich" DNA hybridization, enzyme-modified NPs were brought close to the microbead surface and a fluorescent label or an enzyme-

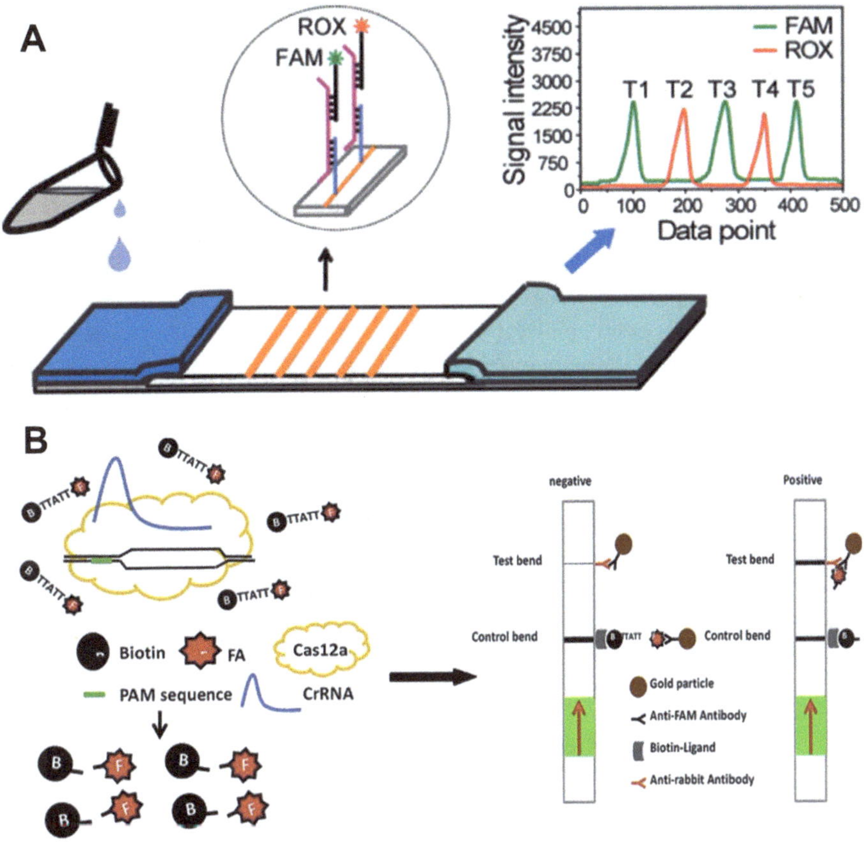

Fig. 6.2 (**a**) Schematic of lateral flow strip based detection of 14 different HPV strains using fluorescent dyes ROX and FAM. Reprinted (adapted) with permission from [38], Copyright (2014) American Chemical Society (**b**) Schematic of lateral flow strip based detection of HPV-16 in plasma samples by utilizing the Cas12a protein [40]. (Copyrights Received)

modified NPs with secondary HPV DNA probes were introduced in a microchannel and the fluorescent signals were measured to quantify the target HPV DNA.

There are also several studies reporting that fluorescent probes labeled with various fluorophores have been used in the lateral flow assay for HPV DNA detection [38–41]. In addition to typical lateral flow devices which use a different strip for each HPV type, Xu et al. have developed a multiplex detection system by fabricating a strip with multiple test lines (14 probes), each coated with a probe specific for a particular HPV strain and two fluorescently labeled capture probes (FAM and ROX) that are designed to bind to alternate test lines (Fig. 6.2a). Thence, fluorescence readout at the different test lines allows for multiplexed detection of PCR amplified samples with minimal cross-reactivity and a detection limit of up to 100 copies of HPV/μL of the sample [38]. A rather novel approach using the biological molecular scissors—CRISPR-Cas has also been applied to lateral flow strips for HPV detection. The Cas12a protein can not only recognize the presence of HPV16 and HPV18 DNA in the presence of a suitable guide RNA but can also cleave other ssDNA in its immediate environment as collaterals. Exploiting its unique nature, Tsou et al. have developed a lateral flow strip utilizing a FAM-biotin reporter system, gold nanoparticle tagged antibodies as in Fig. 6.2b [40]. The unique design allows for visualization of the test band only in the presence of HPV 16 in plasma samples without DNA isolation and PCR amplification, with a detection limit of 0.24 fM. As lateral flow strips are disposable, simple to use, and can be used for rapid analysis of real samples containing HPV, they are an easy and effective method for genotyping HPV in local hospitals.

However, most of these fluorescence sensors still need target amplification process to get reliable fluorescence signal from ultra-small concentration of targets in real samples. An alternative solution to such a problem is signal amplification instead of target amplification as proposed by Chan et al. While adopting the typical DNA hybridization setup using a probe and a biotin modified target DNA, instead of using any commercial fluorescent molecule, they propose the attachment of fluorescein diacetate crystals (precursor) to the hybridized complex via biotin. The resulting fluorescence obtained upon solubilization of the crystals was found to significantly improve the sensitivity of the output signal up to 147 times when compared to the use of commercial fluorescent molecules [42].

6.3 Colorimetric Biosensor

Colorimetric biosensors are devices that are capable to detect certain target molecules with naked eyes through color changes without the need of complicated instruments [43–47]. Plasmonic nanomaterials such as gold nanoparticles (AuNPs) and silver nanoparticles (AgNPs) are generally used as probes in colorimetric sensors. For instance, dispersed AuNPs with size smaller than 20 nm have red color because of the LSPR existing at the wavelength close to 520 nm. However, once AuNPs become aggregated, significant redshift of the LSPR occurs with the color change occurring from red to blue. Since AuNPs can easily be functionalized with biomolecules, such as DNA or proteins through Au-thiol chemistry, aggregation of AuNPs mediated by the biological interaction occurring between complementary DNA molecules or antibody and antigen can happen. Thence, colorimetric sensors exploiting the above principle have also been adapted for the detection of different types of HPV DNA [48, 49]. A classic example of this has been demonstrated by Azizah et al. where they have reported the development of a DNA sensor for the detection of HPV-16 [50]. In the presence of the PCR amplified target DNA, the color of the probe DNA immobilized AuNP solution turns from red to purple due to the aggregation of AuNPs in support of the hypothesis mentioned earlier. In addition, another widely adopted DNA amplification technique-loop-mediated isothermal amplification (LAMP) has also been used to detect HPV DNA by adopting the same principle. The study reports a detection limit of 10–1000 copies of HPV-18 with a reaction time of 20 min to visualize the presence of the target in the cervical tissue sample with the naked eye [51].

While the former studies involved the direct detection of HPV DNA via typical aggregation of AuNPs without the use of an indicator/dye, other studies have also focused on incorporating dyes since a more significant color change can be observed in their presence, improving their practicality for naked eye based detection. Lue et al. reported that LAMP-AuNP colorimetric assay can be used for rapid and simple detection of HPV DNA strands with the naked eye using hydroxy naphthol blue as an indicator [49]. Along similar lines, a "smart connected pathogen tracer" has been developed by Yin *et.al* for the real-time detection of HPV-16 in clinical vaginal swab samples. Instead of using hydroxy naphthol blue as in the previous study, this study utilizes Erichrome-black T (EBT) as an indicator to identify the by-products of a non-buffered LAMP reaction, resulting in three times higher sensitivity when compared to HNB and an appreciable limit of detection of 100 copies HPV DNA per sample [52]. In the presence of the HPV target, PP_i^{4-} (a by-product of LAMP) reacts with the Mg^{2+} bound to EBT resulting in the formation of $Mg_2P_2O_7$ color change from red to blue as the EBT is released, which has been successfully monitored using a Hue analyzer [53]. Instead of EBT, Daskou et al. have used a pH indicator—phenol red to analyze whether LAMP proceeds or not. The basic principle behind this being the fact that there is a liberation of protons as a by-product of LAMP resulting in the reduction in pH of the solution and thus a color change from bright pink to yellow is observed, in the presence of the target. The study claims that this technique yields sensitivity and specificity of 100%, respectively, with the ability to detect with the naked eye as low as 10 copies of HPV-16/HPV-18 per test [54].

As opposed to target amplification via PCR/LAMP as discussed earlier, signal amplification is an alternative strategy to eliminate complex instrumentation and reduce the assay time. In pursuit of this goal, Persano et al. have developed a DNAzyme based double isothermal amplification system (Fig. 6.3) which enables enzymatic recycling of target yielding a significant signal amplification [55]. In the presence of the target (HPV-16), it binds to the magnetic nanoparticles via the RNA probes conjugated with DNAzyme (Horseradish peroxidase mimic). Upon addition of RNaseH which cleaves RNA in a DNA-RNA hybrid, the DNAzyme is released. In the presence of the ABTS (substrate for the DNAzyme), a deep green color is observed in a concentration-dependent manner (0.1 nM- 1μM) which is noticeable with the naked eye (Fig. 6.3a). A similar DNAzyme based signal amplification strategy has also been adopted to develop a ratiometric fluorescent sensor for the detection of HPV-16 using chameleon fluorescent DNA templated silver nanoclusters [56].

While DNAzymes mimic enzyme activity, enzyme-based cascading activity coupled with a microfluidic setup (enzyme-assisted nanocomplexes for visual identification of nucleic acids (enVision)) have also been directly applied towards detection of HPV [57]. In the presence of the target DNA, the otherwise inactive Taq DNA polymerase (bound by aptamer) becomes active which promotes the

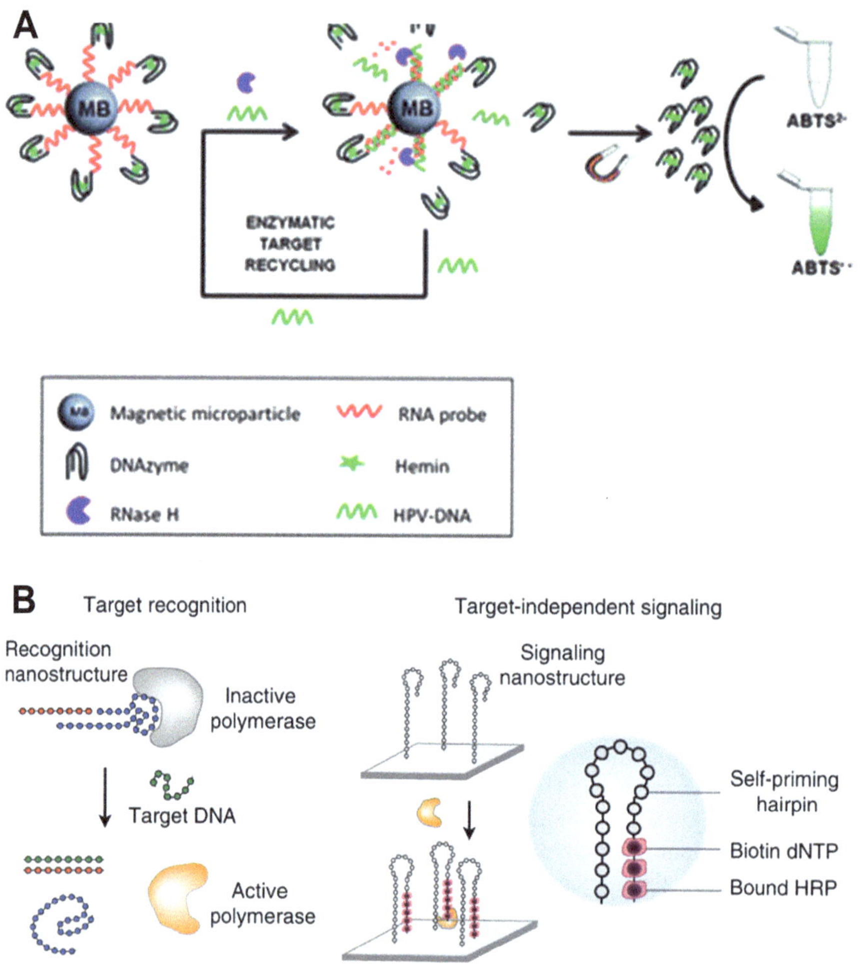

Fig. 6.3 (**a**) Working principle for the colorimetric detection of HPV-16 using DNAzymes bound to magnetic microparticles [55]. (**b**) Principle of the enzyme-cascading activity-based colorimetric sensor for the detection of HPV 16/18 [57]. (Copyrights Received)

extension of the self-primed hairpin structure by incorporation of biotin-labeled nucleotides. Upon incubation with HRP, a target DNA concentration-dependent variation in brown color is observed with the naked eye in the presence of HRP substrate (Fig. 6.3b). Since the complete process is coupled to a microfluidic setup (modularity) and particularly well-designed enzymes are used (specificity, sensitivity), detection limit of up to 7.2 amol has been achieved when the samples are subjected to asymmetric amplification followed by smartphone camera-based processing with a total assay time of only 30 min (excluding asymmetric PCR).

In addition to DNA, peptide nucleic acid (PNA) is also an attractive probe for HPV detection since they have a higher hybridization efficiency to form PNA-DNA hybrids compared to their DNA counterparts and alleviate the need for immobilization of DNA onto the NPs as PNA is charged neutral and can spontaneously bind to NPs resulting in their aggregation. Exploiting these advantages, a paper-based disposable DNA sensor for HPV-16 has been developed by Teengam et al. [58]. In the presence of the target DNA, aggregated AgNPs (PNA bound) are redispersed due to hybridization between the PNA probe and the target resulting in a visual color change from red to yellow with a detection limit of 1.03 nM.

6.4 Conclusion

It is thence clear that in terms of DNA based optical sensors for cervical cancer, the predominant target is the detection of HPV DNA via hybridization reactions. However, these techniques require relatively large amount of purified DNA via PCR/LAMP and lot of time for analysis. Plausible future directions include the utilization of DNA aptamers that can directly bind to either the viral capsid or a virus-infected cell [59] for quantitative detection of the number of viral particles that can further be extrapolated to the stage of cancer. Moreover, resulting color changes of colorimetric assays are generally not clearly recognized with the naked eye up to certain concentration of HPV target DNAs and thence require complex instrumentation limiting their practical applicability. Coupling of optical methods with other detection strategies, for instance, electrochemiluminescence [60] can further improve the sensitivity without compromising on the selectivity by utilizing the unique advantages of each of the techniques. Thus, further research is needed to develop alternative methods, which are a simple, fast, highly reliable, and easy to handle at low cost for practical use of the colorimetric sensors for the detection of HPV.

Declaration of Competing Interest The authors declare no conflicts of interest.

Acknowledgements Authors are grateful to the Ministry of Human Resource Development, Government of India for the financial support through *Scheme for Promotion of Academic and Research Collaboration* (*SPARC*) project "SPARC/2018-2019/P402/SL". We also acknowledge the support received from the National Research Foundation (NRF) of Korea for the Basic Science Research Program funded by the Ministry of Education (NRF-2019R1A6A1A03033215). We are grateful to SASTRA Deemed University, India and SKKU, South Korea for providing infrastructural support.

References

1. Cooper MA (2002) Optical biosensors in drug discovery. Nat Rev Drug Discov 1:515–528. https://doi.org/10.1038/nrd838

2. Damborský P, Švitel J, Katrlík J (2016) Optical biosensors. Essays Biochem 60:91–100. https://doi.org/10.1042/ebc20150010
3. Heo JH, Cho HH, Lee JH (2014) Surfactant-free nanoparticle–DNA complexes with ultrahigh stability against salt for environmental and biological sensing. Analyst 139:5936–5944. https://doi.org/10.1039/C4AN01271B
4. Heo JH, Yi GS, Lee BS, Cho HH, Lee JW, Lee JH (2016) A significant enhancement of color transition from an on–off type achromatic colorimetric nanosensor for highly sensitive multi-analyte detection with the naked eye. Nanoscale 8:18341–18351. https://doi.org/10.1039/C6NR05919H
5. Shao B, Xiao Z (2020) Recent achievements in exosomal biomarkers detection by nanomaterials-based optical biosensors - a review. Anal Chim Acta 1114:74–84. https://doi.org/10.1016/j.aca.2020.02.041
6. Dickinson TA, White J, Kauer JS, Walt DR (1996) A chemical-detecting system based on a cross-reactive optical sensor array. Nature 382:697–700. https://doi.org/10.1038/382697a0
7. Holtz JH, Asher SA (1997) Polymerized colloidal crystal hydrogel films as intelligent chemical sensing materials. Nature 389:829–832. https://doi.org/10.1038/39834
8. Homola J, Yee SS, Gauglitz G (1999) Surface plasmon resonance sensors: review. Sensors Actuators B Chem 54:3–15. https://doi.org/10.1016/S0925-4005(98)00321-9
9. Rosenstein JK, Wanunu M, Merchant CA, Drndic M, Shepard KL (2012) Integrated nanopore sensing platform with sub-microsecond temporal resolution. Nat Methods 9:487–492. https://doi.org/10.1038/nmeth.1932
10. Miles BN, Ivanov AP, Wilson KA, Doğan F, Japrung D, Edel JB (2013) Single molecule sensing with solid-state nanopores: novel materials, methods, and applications. Chem Soc Rev 42:15–28. https://doi.org/10.1039/c2cs35286a
11. Khanna Vinod K (2008) New-generation nano-engineered biosensors, enabling nanotechnologies and nanomaterials. Sens Rev 28:39–45. https://doi.org/10.1108/02602280810850017
12. Pilolli R, Monaci L, Visconti A (2013) Advances in biosensor development based on integrating nanotechnology and applied to food-allergen management. TrAC Trends Anal Chem 47:12–26. https://doi.org/10.1016/j.trac.2013.02.005
13. Huang X, Liu Y, Yung B, Xiong Y, Chen X (2017) Nanotechnology-enhanced no-wash biosensors for in vitro diagnostics of cancer. ACS Nano 11:5238–5292. https://doi.org/10.1021/acsnano.7b02618
14. Dhathathreyan A (2011) Real-time monitoring of Invertase activity immobilized in Nanoporous Aluminum oxide. J Phys Chem B 115:6678–6682. https://doi.org/10.1021/jp1122085
15. Hotta K, Yamaguchi A, Teramae N (2012) Nanoporous waveguide sensor with optimized Nanoarchitectures for highly sensitive label-free biosensing. ACS Nano 6:1541–1547. https://doi.org/10.1021/nn204494z
16. Heo JH, Kim K-I, Cho HH, Lee JW, Lee BS, Yoon S, Park KJ, Lee S, Kim J, Whang D et al. (2015) Ultrastable-stealth large gold nanoparticles with DNA directed biological functionality. Langmuir 31:13773–13782. https://doi.org/10.1021/acs.langmuir.5b03534
17. Celik M, Altuntas S, Buyukserin F (2018) Fabrication of nanocrater-decorated anodic aluminum oxide membranes as substrates for reproducibly enhanced SERS signals. Sensors Actuators B Chem 255:2871–2877. https://doi.org/10.1016/j.snb.2017.09.105
18. Park J, Kim J, Kim S-Y, Cheong WH, Jang J, Park Y-G, Na K, Kim Y-T, Heo JH, Lee CY et al. (2018) Soft, smart contact lenses with integrations of wireless circuits, glucose sensors, and displays. Sci Adv 4:eaap9841. https://doi.org/10.1126/sciadv.aap9841
19. Lizard G, Chignol MC, Souchier C, Roignot P, Chardonnet Y, Schmitt D (1998) Detection of low copy numbers of HPV DNA by fluorescent in situ hybridization combined with confocal microscopy as an alternative to in situ polymerase chain reaction. J Virol Methods 72:15–25. https://doi.org/10.1016/S0166-0934(98)00008-1

20. Lee JH, Yigit MV, Mazumdar D, Lu Y (2010) Molecular diagnostic and drug delivery agents based on aptamer-nanomaterial conjugates. Adv Drug Deliv Rev 62:592–605. https://doi.org/10.1016/j.addr.2010.03.003
21. Bauch M, Toma K, Toma M, Zhang Q, Dostalek J (2014) Plasmon-enhanced fluorescence biosensors: a review. Plasmonics 9:781–799. https://doi.org/10.1007/s11468-013-9660-5
22. Dodeigne C, Thunus L, Lejeune R (2000) Chemiluminescence as diagnostic tool. A review. Talanta 51:415–439. https://doi.org/10.1016/S0039-9140(99)00294-5
23. Frías I, Avelino K, Silva R, Andrade C, Oliveira M (2015) Trends in biosensors for HPV: identification and diagnosis. J Sensors 2015:1–16. https://doi.org/10.1155/2015/913640
24. Saylan Y, Erdem Ö, Ünal S, Denizli A (2019) An alternative medical diagnosis method: biosensors for virus detection. Biosensors 9:65. https://doi.org/10.3390/bios9020065
25. Wang W, Pang D-W, Tang H-W (2014) Sensitive multiplexed DNA detection using silica nanoparticles as the target capturing platform. Talanta 128:263–267. https://doi.org/10.1016/j.talanta.2014.05.011
26. Ricco R, Meneghello A, Enrichi F (2011) Signal enhancement in DNA microarray using dye doped silica nanoparticles: application to human papilloma virus (HPV) detection. Biosens Bioelectron 26:2761–2765. https://doi.org/10.1016/j.bios.2010.10.024
27. Peng X, Zhang Y, Lu D, Guo Y, Guo S (2019) Ultrathin Ti3C2 nanosheets based "off-on" fluorescent nanoprobe for rapid and sensitive detection of HPV infection. Sensors Actuators B Chem 286:222–229. https://doi.org/10.1016/j.snb.2019.01.158
28. Xiang D-S, Zeng G-P, He Z-K (2011) Magnetic microparticle-based multiplexed DNA detection with biobarcoded quantum dot probes. Biosens Bioelectron 26:4405–4410. https://doi.org/10.1016/j.bios.2011.04.051
29. Yu-Hong W, Rui C, Ding L (2011) A quantum dots and superparamagnetic nanoparticle-based method for the detection of HPV DNA. Nanoscale Res Lett 6:461. https://doi.org/10.1186/1556-276X-6-461
30. Shamsipur M, Nasirian V, Mansouri K, Barati A, Veisi-Raygani A, Kashanian S (2017) A highly sensitive quantum dots-DNA nanobiosensor based on fluorescence resonance energy transfer for rapid detection of nanomolar amounts of human papillomavirus 18. J Pharm Biomed Anal 136:140–147. https://doi.org/10.1016/j.jpba.2017.01.002
31. Huang C-C, Yang Z, Lee K-H, Chang H-T (2007) Synthesis of highly fluorescent gold nanoparticles for sensing mercury(II). Angew Chem Int Ed 46:6824–6828. https://doi.org/10.1002/anie.200700803
32. Ray PC, Darbha GK, Ray A, Hardy W, Walker J (2007) A gold-nanoparticle-based fluorescence resonance energy transfer probe for multiplexed hybridization detection: accurate identification of bio-agents DNA. Nanotechnology 18:375504. https://doi.org/10.1088/0957-4484/18/37/375504
33. He S, Song B, Li D, Zhu C, Qi W, Wen Y, Wang L, Song S, Fang H, Fan C (2010) A graphene nanoprobe for rapid, sensitive, and multicolor fluorescent DNA analysis. Adv Funct Mater 20:453–459. https://doi.org/10.1002/adfm.200901639
34. Tan C, Yu P, Hu Y, Chen J, Huang Y, Cai Y, Luo Z, Li B, Lu Q, Wang L et al. (2015) High-yield exfoliation of ultrathin two-dimensional ternary chalcogenide nanosheets for highly sensitive and selective fluorescence DNA sensors. J Am Chem Soc 137:10430–10436. https://doi.org/10.1021/jacs.5b06982
35. Zhang W, Li S, Li X, Liu M, Cui T, Fu H, Yang M, Zhong W, Xu B, Yue W (2020) PEG-PtS2 nanosheet-based fluorescence biosensor for label-free human papillomavirus genotyping. Microchim Acta 187:408. https://doi.org/10.1007/s00604-020-04383-8
36. Zhang H, Liu L, Li C-W, Fu H, Chen Y, Yang M (2011) Multienzyme-nanoparticles amplification for sensitive virus genotyping in microfluidic microbeads array using Au nanoparticle probes and quantum dots as labels. Biosens Bioelectron 29:89–96. https://doi.org/10.1016/j.bios.2011.07.074

37. Yue W, Zou H, Jin Q, Li C-W, Xu T, Fu H, Tzang LCH, Sun H, Zhao J, Yang M (2014) Single layer linear array of microbeads for multiplexed analysis of DNA and proteins. Biosens Bioelectron 54:297–305. https://doi.org/10.1016/j.bios.2013.10.034
38. Xu Y, Liu Y, Wu Y, Xia X, Liao Y, Li Q (2014) Fluorescent probe-based lateral flow assay for multiplex nucleic acid detection. Anal Chem 86:5611–5614. https://doi.org/10.1021/ac5010458
39. Kumvongpin R, Jearanaikoon P, Wilailuckana C, Sae-Ung N, Prasongdee P, Daduang S, Wongsena M, Boonsiri P, Kiatpathomchai W, Swangvaree SS et al. (2017) Detection assay for HPV16 and HPV18 by loopmediated isothermal amplification with lateral flow dipstick tests. Mol Med Rep 15:3203–3209. https://doi.org/10.3892/mmr.2017.6370
40. Tsou JH, Leng Q, Jiang F (2019) A CRISPR test for detection of circulating nuclei acids. Transl Oncol 12:1566–1573. https://doi.org/10.1016/j.tranon.2019.08.011
41. Yang Z, Yi C, Lv S, Sheng Y, Wen W, Zhang X, Wang S (2019) Development of a lateral flow strip biosensor based on copper oxide nanoparticles for rapid and sensitive detection of HPV16 DNA. Sensors Actuators B Chem 285:326–332. https://doi.org/10.1016/j.snb.2019.01.056
42. Chan CP, Tzang LC, Sin KK, Ji SL, Cheung KY, Tam TK, Yang MM, Renneberg R, Seydack M (2007) Biofunctional organic nanocrystals for quantitative detection of pathogen deoxyribonucleic acid. Anal Chim Acta 584:7–11. https://doi.org/10.1016/j.aca.2006.11.025
43. Heo JH, Kim K-I, Lee MH, Lee JH (2013) Stability of a gold nanoparticle-DNA system in seawater. J Nanosci Nanotechnol 13:7254–7258. https://doi.org/10.1166/jnn.2013.8101
44. Heo JH, Cho HH, Lee JW, Lee JH (2014) Achromatic–chromatic colorimetric sensors for on–off type detection of analytes. Analyst 139:6486–6493. https://doi.org/10.1039/C4AN01645A
45. Sabela M, Balme S, Bechelany M, Janot J-M, Bisetty K (2017) A review of gold and silver nanoparticle-based colorimetric sensing assays. Adv Eng Mater 19:1700270. https://doi.org/10.1002/adem.201700270
46. Aldewachi H, Chalati T, Woodroofe MN, Bricklebank N, Sharrack B, Gardiner P (2018) Gold nanoparticle-based colorimetric biosensors. Nanoscale 10:18–33. https://doi.org/10.1039/C7NR06367A
47. Cho HH, Kim SJ, Jafry AT, Lee B, Heo JH, Yoon S, Jeong SH, Kang S-I, Lee JH, Lee J (2019) A paper-based platform for long-term deposition of nanoparticles with exceptional redispersibility, stability, and functionality. Part Part Syst Charact 36:1800483. https://doi.org/10.1002/ppsc.201800483
48. Chen S, Lin K, Tang C, Peng S, Chuang Y, Lin Y, Wang J, Lin C (2009) Optical detection of human papillomavirus type 16 and type 18 by sequence sandwich hybridization with oligonucleotide-functionalized au nanoparticles. IEEE Trans Nanobioscience 8:120–131. https://doi.org/10.1109/TNB.2008.2011733
49. Luo L, Nie K, Yang M-J, Wang M, Li J, Zhang C, Liu H-T, Ma X-J (2011) Visual detection of high-risk human papillomavirus genotypes 16, 18, 45, 52, and 58 by loop-mediated isothermal amplification with hydroxynaphthol blue dye. J Clin Microbiol 49:3545–3550. https://doi.org/10.1128/JCM.00930-11
50. Azizah N, Hashim U, Gopinath SCB, Nadzirah S (2017) A direct detection of human papillomavirus 16 genomic DNA using gold nanoprobes. Int J Biol Macromol 94:571–575. https://doi.org/10.1016/j.ijbiomac.2016.10.060
51. Kumvongpin R, Jearanaikool P, Wilailuckana C, Sae-Ung N, Prasongdee P, Daduang S, Wongsena M, Boonsiri P, Kiatpathomchai W, Swangvaree SS et al. (2016) High sensitivity, loop-mediated isothermal amplification combined with colorimetric gold-nanoparticle probes for visual detection of high risk human papillomavirus genotypes 16 and 18. J Virol Methods 234:90–95. https://doi.org/10.1016/j.jviromet.2016.04.008
52. Yin K, Pandian V, Kadimisetty K, Zhang X, Ruiz C, Cooper K, Liu C (2020) Real-time colorimetric quantitative molecular detection of infectious diseases on smartphone-based diagnostic platform. Sci Rep 10:9009. https://doi.org/10.1038/s41598-020-65899-w
53. Yin K, Pandian V, Kadimisetty K, Ruiz C, Cooper K, You J, Liu C (2019) Synergistically enhanced colorimetric molecular detection using smart cup: a case for instrument-free

HPV-associated cancer screening. Theranostics 9:2637–2645. https://doi.org/10.7150/thno.32224
54. Daskou M, Tsakogiannis D, Dimitriou TG, Amoutzias GD, Mossialos D, Kottaridi C, Gartzonika C, Markoulatos P (2019) WarmStart colorimetric LAMP for the specific and rapid detection of HPV16 and HPV18 DNA. J Virol Methods 270:87–94. https://doi.org/10.1016/j.jviromet.2019.04.023
55. Persano S, Valentini P, Kim JH, Pompa PP (2013) Colorimetric detection of human papilloma virus by double isothermal amplification. Chem Commun (Camb) 49:10605–10607. https://doi.org/10.1039/c3cc45459b
56. Yuan Y, Ma Y, Luo L, Wang Q, Huang J, Liu J, Yang X, Wang K (2019) Ratiometric determination of human papillomavirus-16 DNA by using fluorescent DNA-templated silver nanoclusters and hairpin-blocked DNAzyme-assisted cascade amplification. Mikrochim Acta 186:613. https://doi.org/10.1007/s00604-019-3732-y
57. Ho NRY, Lim GS, Sundah NR, Lim D, Loh TP, Shao H (2018) Visual and modular detection of pathogen nucleic acids with enzyme-DNA molecular complexes. Nat Commun 9:3238. https://doi.org/10.1038/s41467-018-05733-0
58. Teengam P, Siangproh W, Tuantranont A, Vilaivan T, Chailapakul O, Henry CS (2017) Multiplex paper-based colorimetric DNA sensor using Pyrrolidinyl peptide nucleic acid-induced AgNPs aggregation for detecting MERS-CoV, MTB, and HPV oligonucleotides. Anal Chem 89:5428–5435. https://doi.org/10.1021/acs.analchem.7b00255
59. Bamrungsap S, Treetong A, Apiwat C, Wuttikhun T, Dharakul T (2015) SERS-fluorescence dual mode nanotags for cervical cancer detection using aptamers conjugated to gold-silver nanorods. Microchim Acta 183:249–256. https://doi.org/10.1007/s00604-015-1639-9
60. Nie Y, Zhang X, Zhang Q, Liang Z, Ma Q, Su X (2020) A novel high efficient electrochemiluminescence sensor based on reductive Cu(I) particles catalyzed Zn-doped MoS2 QDs for HPV 16 DNA determination. Biosens Bioelectron 160:112217. https://doi.org/10.1016/j.bios.2020.112217

Other Biosensors for Cervical Cancer Detection

7

Raghavv Raghavender Suresh, Priyannth Ramasami Sundhar Baabu, John Bosco Balaguru Rayappan, and Arockia Jayalatha JBB

Abstract

Although electrochemical and optical biosensors have taken over the bulk of the scientific literature and the commercial market, it is necessary for the scientific audience to be exposed to other sensing methodologies associated with cervical cancer diagnosis. Subsequently, the scientific principles behind different transduction platforms for biosensing, ranging from the gold-standard molecular biology technique of polymerase chain reaction (PCR) to the game changing nano-thermometry, are discussed in this chapter. Further, works pertaining to the detection of biomarkers and the diagnosis of cervical cancer using these platforms have been elucidated. Apart from the prementioned techniques, scientific principles and reports of cervical cancer diagnosis pertaining to vibrational spectroscopic methods, mechanical transducers, and field effect transistor (FET) based transducers are discussed here. Also, challenges associated with each

R. R. Suresh · P. R. S. Baabu
Centre for Nanotechnology and Advanced Biomaterials (CeNTAB), SASTRA Deemed University, Thanjavur, Tamil Nadu, India

School of Chemical and Biotechnology, SASTRA Deemed University, Thanjavur, Tamil Nadu, India

J. B. B. Rayappan
Centre for Nanotechnology and Advanced Biomaterials (CeNTAB), School of Electrical and Electronics Engineering, SASTRA Deemed University, Thanjavur, Tamil Nadu, India

A. J. JBB (✉)
School of Electrical and Electronics Engineering, SASTRA Deemed University, Thanjavur, Tamil Nadu, India
e-mail: arockiajayalatha@eee.sastra.edu

J. B. B. Rayappan, J. H. Lee (eds.), *Biomarkers and Biosensors for Cervical Cancer Diagnosis*, https://doi.org/10.1007/978-981-16-2586-2_7

sensing methodology are critically analysed. Further, novel optical sensors that have made it into the commercial market are discussed selectively. We believe that such constructive discussions could aid the readers in discerning the shortfalls associated with the commercialisation of different biosensing techniques.

Keywords

Nanothermometry · Vibrational spectroscopy · PCR · Piezoelectric sensors · Cervical cancer · HeLa

7.1 Introduction

Cervical cancer detection is paramount, considering the fact that it is one among the few cancers, which, when identified early, could effectively increase the survival probability of the patient. Hence, for this cause, variegated strategies and methodologies have been employed with the help of biotechnology and nanotechnology, predominantly. Earlier chapters discussed about the design, fabrication and utility of electrochemical and optical DNA biosensors, in detailed terms. This chapter would bring under its umbrella the other kinds of biosensors that have been designed, fabricated and utilised for cervical cancer detection. These are mechanical biosensors, PCR-based biosensors, thermal based biosensors, spectroscopy-based biosensors, electric biosensors and other optical biosensors.

7.2 Temperature Based Detection

The eukaryotic cell may be envisaged as a factory with each organelle in this highly compartmentalised entity performing specific functions and subsequently possessing varying energy needs. As a consequence, the intracellular temperature distribution varies, for instance, mitochondria, the power-house of the cell, is reported to be warm, centrosome dividing locations and the milieu around the nucleus generates heat [1]. Rapid cell proliferation, a well-defined characteristic of cancer cells, may cause varied energy utilisation in the cell and hence the intracellular temperature distribution profile may vary in cancer cells. Further, reports suggest tumour cells possess higher temperatures than normal cells [2]. Conversely, hyperthermia is a preferred adjuvant therapy and is used alongside other conventional therapies such as chemotherapy and radiotherapy. This treatment technique induces apoptosis, inhibits DNA repair mechanisms in hyperthermia targeted cells and is promising towards treating radiotherapy resistant cancer cells. Further, hyperthermia triggers growth of heat shock protein - 70 (HSP-70) on targeted cells and results in activation of natural killer cells and production of cytotoxins to facilitate tumour cell annihilation [3, 4]. In the case of cervical cancer patients, Burchardt and Roszak [5] reported hyperthermia to aid their survival [5]. However, even in the case of local hyperthermia, this method is limited by its inability to confine heating effects only to the tumour regions and hence, the plausibility to affect its neighbouring tissue regions is very prevalent [6, 7]. Such unintended effects can be avoided by appropriate choice of heating and ensuring that the heat is localised in tumour regions. The pre-mentioned scenario of temperature differences in tumour cells and the necessity to prevent off-targeting in hyperthermia therapy subsequently demands an effective strategy to monitor temperature variations within and around the tumour environment. Considering these aspects, intracellular temperature measurement-based strategies and thermal imaging studies are discussed in this section.

7.2.1 Nanothermometry

Nanothermometry is intended to measure the local temperature changes with sub-micrometre spatial resolution and is useful towards probing intracellular dynamics, organelle [8] and chemical dependent thermogenesis [9, 10] and hence finds immense prospects in biomedicine [11–14]. This technique can be broadly categorised into three groups: electrical, mechanical and optical. Electrical nanothermometry utilises conventional thermocouple and thermistor-based concepts where the changes in voltage and resistance (respectively) are characteristic of temperature measurements [15]. On the other hand, microfabrication technologies have been appropriately leveraged for fabricating submicron-sized thermal sensors, known as scanning thermal microscopy, which is like atomic force microscopy (AFM). Here, the tip of the thermocouple probe is in contact with the surface and scanned to obtain a 2-dimensional (2D) image. For instance, Wang et al. [16] reported a thermocouple based nanothermometer that provided highly accurate thermal signal values with very good time-scale resolution characteristics [16]. Mechanical nanothermometry involves a bimaterial containing a micro-cantilever. Owing to differences in mechanical properties in different segments of the probe, there is a significant deflection corresponding to temperature changes in the environment, which can be used for temperature monitoring. However, both of the techniques are limited by their ability to obtain only 2D surface images. Furthermore, the physical contact between the probe tip and the surface may incur complex heat flux transfer while the cost of fabricating these sensors is also high [17]. Interferometry and reflectance-based analysis involve measuring changes pertaining to refractive index and surface thickness. The latter values, in turn, change with temperature fluctuations and are indicative of the temperature profile of the surroundings'. In this regard, the optical nanothermography technique utilises these passive optical parameters to comment on the temperature distribution of the system. However, these techniques are generally used to obtain 2D thermal images of the surface.

Excitation of the outermost valence electrons in an atom to higher, less stable energy levels aids it to liberate the gained energy as heat and light to transit to less excited, more stable ground state energy levels. The light emitted as a result of this process is termed luminescence, and depending on the excitation source, it can be classified into chemiluminescence, bioluminescence, triboluminescence and

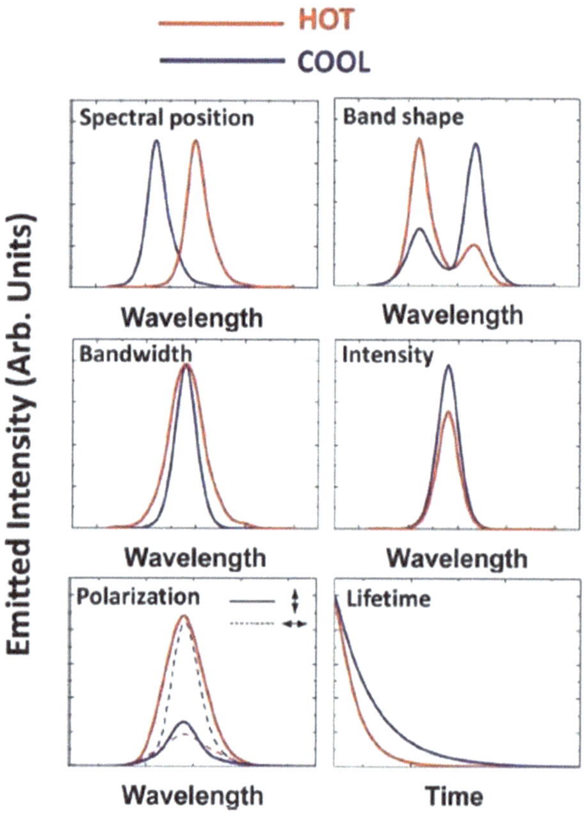

Fig. 7.1 Variations in luminescence with temperature increment (Copyrights received) [19]

photoluminescence. Photoluminescence involves the excitation of a substance by optical radiation and generally results in emission radiation having a higher wavelength than the excitation wavelength. This is known as Stokes emission. The decrease in energy may be attributed to other non-radiative energy losses associated with vibration and heat liberation. Further the radiations emitted are classified based on variations in spin multiplicity, which may occur as a result of excitation of electrons to higher energy levels. If there are no changes in spin multiplicity on excitation, the electron transits to a singlet excited state and returns to the ground state within 10 ns and it is known as fluorescence (allowed transition). Conversely, on reversal of spin multiplicity, the electron occupies the excited triplet state via transition to the ground state is quantum mechanically forbidden. As a result, this causes a delayed emission, which is known as phosphorescence. As mentioned, the emission radiation is dependent on the electronic states, which depend on the temperature of the surroundings. Hence, luminescence measurements can be utilised to analyse the thermal energy distribution of the environment [18].

Luminescence nanothermometry exploits this concept and is analysed based on any of the six parameters shown in Fig. 7.1. (1) **Intensity luminescent nanothermometry**: with changes in temperature, the flux of photons emitted correspondingly decreases and subsequently there is a change in intensity, which is characteristic of temperature distribution. (2) **Band shape luminescence nanothermometry**: With thermal fluctuations, as the spectral lines of luminescence emission are close to one another, the band shape is susceptible to undergo changes, thereby indicating temperature variations in the environment. (3) **Spectral luminescence nanothermometry**: Spectral line positions depend on the energy levels of electronic states and are characteristic of the refractive index & inter-atomic distance in a material. With variations in temperature, spectral line positions vary correspondingly and are hence used for temperature distribution analysis. (4) **Polarisation luminescence nanothermometry**: involves measuring the ratio of parallel and perpendicular polarisation components relative to incident polarisation direction whose ratio is largely influenced by the Brownian motion of the luminescent particles. Further, Brownian motion is largely dependent on the temperature profile of the surroundings. Hence, the polarisation anisotropy values obtained from the ratio of the parallel and perpendicular components may be exploited to comment on the thermal fluctuations of the environment. (5) **Bandwidth luminescence nanothermometry**: phonon density largely depends on the temperature fluctuations in the environment and further influences the spectral bandwidth, hence it may be leveraged for thermal profile analysis. (6) **Lifetime luminescence nanothermometry**: utilises the decay probability of radiations which decreases with phonon assisted energy transfer, where phonon generation is largely dependent on thermal fluctuations, which can be used for temperature distribution analysis. Luminescence nanothermometry offers very high thermal sensitivity characteristics. With improvements in nanoparticle synthesis techniques, surface functionalization and dispersion methodologies, this nanothermometry technique may offer very high spatial resolution for thermal sensing. [19]. Hence, this section encompasses a discussion of luminescence nanothermometry and its prospects for cervical cancer detection.

Fluorescent protein based nanothermometers, which can be genetically encoded, facilitate organelle targeting. However, these probes have low thermal sensitivity [20]. Albeit, organic fluorescent dyes possess considerable intracellular targeting ability and thermal sensitivity, photobleaching issues exist [20]. Fluorescent nanogels, owing to their large size and low hydrophilicity, find little utility in intracellular temperature sensing [21]. However, recent works by Okabe et al. [22], pertaining to reducing the size of nanogels and modifying their surface with hydrophilic residues, have rendered them useful for intracellular temperature measurements [22]. Inorganic quantum dot (QD) based nanothermometers exhibit significant spatial localisation [23]. However, photobleaching of QDs has been reported [24]. Upconverting nanoparticles (UCNPs) possess excellent photostability, excitability in the NIR range and are used in biological applications [25]. Owing to their idiosyncratic luminescence properties, a brief description of UCNPs is included here.

UCNPs constitute a host material, an activator and a sensitiser. An ideal host material should have low phonon energies so that the non-radiative energy loss does not hinder the radiative processes which may reduce its efficiency. This may be attributed to the fact that "phonons", quantised vibrational waves of the lattice in interaction with photons, result in "Anti-Stokes Raman Scattering", which is much weaker. Hence, the host material is chosen in the purview of having a low phonon lattice energy. Commonly, inorganic molecules are used. Although salts of heavy halides like Br^- & Cl^- have lower phonon energies, they are hygroscopic and hence not chemically stable. Conversely, oxide-based inorganic materials offer high chemical stability, but the high lattice phonon energies affect their upconversion efficiency. In this context, fluoride based inorganic salts are popularly used and are chemically stable and possess lower phonon energies. Reports suggest covalent host materials result in increased electron–phonon coupling and hence ionic host materials are preferred [26]. Optically active long-lived excited states are more preferred for upconverting systems. Forbidden transitions facilitate such longevity and hence lanthanides, owing to the presence of 4f orbitals are used in UCNPs. Elements present in the middle of lanthanides are reported to have optimal shielding owing to the presence of 5s and 5p orbitals, experience lanthanide contraction and hence do not participate in interaction with the environment or with phonons. The absence of interaction with the neighbouring environment prevents crystal field splitting, i.e. breaking of degeneracy of orbitals, and offers a large number of electronic excited states with similar energy within the forbital. This facilitates f-f transitions, which are forbidden according to the Laporte Selection rules and hence offers long-lived excited states, thereby augmenting the upconversion characteristics. Lower concentrations of activator ions are used and optimum distance between these ions is ensured to prevent cross-relaxation. Sensitiser ions have a high cross-sectional area for IR radiations and have energy level differences like activatorions, promoting energy transfer upconversion [27].

UCNPs have been utilised for temperature monitoring in HeLa, cervical cancer cell lines [28]. The work involved solvothermal synthesis of water dispersible $NaYF_4:Er^{3+}$, Yb^{3+} NPs and the ratio of their emission peaks at 525 and 545 nm was seen to be inversely proportional to temperature values. Further, the solution containing UCNPs was irradiated with a 980 nm laser source and thermal images of the temperature distribution profile which revealed temperature gradient were obtained. UCNPs have been reported to be endocytosed by HeLa cells [29], and these cells were incubated in an UCNPs solution. Voltage was applied to a metallic platform setup and the intracellular temperature of the HeLa cells varied quadratically. Transmission optical images for different temperature values (25°C, 35°C and 45°C) revealed changes in cancer cell's morphology, thereby highlighting the work's significance towards single cell temperature measurements and hyperthermia induced cell death [28].

Carbon dots (CDs) exhibit tuneable fluorescence properties, biocompatibility, possess low cytotoxicity and are water dispersible [30]. Macairan et al. [31] reported a CD based fluorescence nanothermometer for intracellular temperature measurements and demonstrated its real-time usability in HeLa cells. The group synthesised dual fluorescing CDs (dCDs) via microwave synthesis which did not agglomerate even upon drying. Excitation of dCDs at 405 nm yielded blue and red emission peaks centred between 370 and 500 nm and 645 and 730 nm, respectively, whereas excitation of dCDs at 640 nm yielded only a red emission peak. Further, the quantum yield for blue and red peaks was reported to be 0.38% and 6.11%, respectively. The blue fluorescence originated from the core of carbon centres, while the red fluorescence was attributed to the fluorophores attached to carbon atoms in CD. For a 640 nm excitation, the intensity of the red emission peak increased linearly with temperature (5–60°C). However, when the dCDs colloidal solution was excited at 405 nm, there was a dip in intensity for blue emission and an increase in intensity for red emission. Cell viability studies were performed by incubating dCDs in HeLa cells for 24 h and the dCD concentration for IC50 of the cell line was reported to be 147.6 μg mL^{-1}. Although excitation of dCDs at 640 nm offers advantages such as greater penetration depth and less scattering, the red emission intensities did not corroborate with the externally induced thermal changes in the HeLa cells. Conversely, the ratio of red to blue emission intensity for excitation at 405 nm increased linearly with increasing temperatures, thus affirming the utility of the ratio-metric approach for temperature sensing. dCDs exhibit advantages such as being thermally stable, exhibiting real-time and reversible fluorescence response. However, owing to excitation at lower wavelengths, which raises autofluorescence issues in biological tissues, it is difficult to translate this work in vivo [31].

Although DNA based nanothermometers possess advantages such as being biocompatible and demonstrating high spatial and temperature sensitivity, they are prone to nuclease mediated degradation and require external transfection agents for their internalisation into cells. To address these limitations, Xie et al. [32] took cues from nature and synthesised a scallop-inspired DNA nanomachine (SDN), which consisted of a molecular beacon (MB) encapsulated in a tetrahedron DNA arrangement. Like the shell of scallops, the tetrahedron architecture protected the MB from its surroundings and further assisted its quick response to an external stimulus. SDN was synthesised using oligonucleotide strands P1, P2, P3 and P4. P3 contained stem-loop MB structure, acceptor and donor dye molecules were attached to P4 that is partially hybridised to P3 strand. Thus, for temperatures greater than melting temperature (T_m - 54°C), the stem-loop structure unfolded and hence the acceptor to donor signal (A/D) decreased, while for temperatures lower than T_m, the tetrahedron structure remained intact and hence significant A/D signals were obtained. For cyclic variations in temperature between 27 and 54°C the SDN demonstrated reliable reusability and reversibility characteristics. SDN responses did not vary with pH, K^+ concentration and the arrangement was nuclease resistant. Furthermore, the (3-(4,5-dimethylthiazol-2-yl)-2,5-diphenyltetrazolium) bromide) assay or MTT assay revealed the SDN to be non-cytotoxic. SDN's real-time usability was probed in HeLa cells, which highlighted SDN's ability to be endocytosed by cells and thus circumventing the need for external transfection agents. Intracellular temperature measurements were performed by exciting the arrangement at 488 nm and corresponding changes in fluorescence values were seen. The ratio-metric fluorescence signals obtained as A/D values attenuated the effects of environment. Further, SDN was used for simultaneous visualisation of the heating area in gold nanorods incubated with HeLa cells, where the nanorods were irradiated by a 980 nm laser for different time intervals and the corresponding fluorescence signals were monitored. This indeed bolsters SDN's usability for intracellular temperature monitoring [32].

Albeit popularly used cadmium or lead based semiconductor crystal QDs exhibit tuneable emission peaks and resistance to variations in pH, they are toxic and hence not preferred for bioimaging applications. Hence, Zhang et al. [33] synthesised non-toxic and highly biocompatible core/shell binary QDs—$CuInS_2/ZnS$ encapsulated in an amphiphilic micelle. Encapsulation by polyoxyethylene stearate (PS), a derivative of polyethylene glycol (PEG), conferred hydrophilicity to QDs and rendered them dispersible in water. A red shift in emission peak was attributed to the interaction of QD-micelle's surface with polar environment, which affected the electron–hole recombination pairs and hence resulted in bandgap variations. Fluorescence intensities were seen to decrease with increasing temperatures. As far as temperature sensitivity was concerned, micelle encapsulated QDs did not show any significant variations from unencapsulated QDs. The QD-micelle structures were repeatedly heated and cooled to 60°C and 0°C and the structures demonstrated very good thermostability and reversibility characteristics. This was attributed to the tight encapsulation and stable interaction between the QD and the micellar assembly. Even at concentrations as high as 300 $\mu g\ mL^{-1}$, the QD-micelles were not toxic to HeLa and prostate cancer cells. Fluorescence measurements using confocal microscopy revealed no significant changes even after exchanging the previously incubated QD solution medium with a new medium, thus indicating no exocytosis of QDs from cells. Further, these QD-micelles were used for in vivo tumour imaging. Here, they exhibited significant intensity changes in physiological temperatures and very good stability in tissue, thus highlighting their usability for real-time bioimaging applications [33].

Intracellular thermal imaging using non-fluorescent techniques such as thermocouples, Raman microscopy and others is indeed in corroboration with the results obtained from fluorescent intracellular nanothermometers. This has in turn ameliorated the reliability of these nanothermometers. However, currently, along with these temperature measurements, studies record other physiological parameters such as mitochondrial depolarisation and the rate of oxygen consumption to bolster the nanothermometer's results [34]. Nevertheless, simultaneous measurements of other physiological parameters by coupling them with intracellular nanothermometry is a stiff task. Hence, in the case of sole utilisation of fluorescence nanothermometry, it is recommended to make multiple measurements and report the average readings [35]. In vivo nanothermometry is still in its primordial stages. Fluorescence nanothermometry is being probed in animal models, especially for photothermal therapy applications, where the materials emit temperature dependent fluorescence. Further, excitation of materials with EM source results in fluorescence emission as well as heat liberation and thus dual purpose of imaging and thermal treatment is being addressed. Owing to greater penetration depth characteristics and minimal auto-florescence in biological tissues, NIR irradiation is preferred. In order to fabricate safer theranostic systems, temperature monitoring and heating strategies can be appropriately decoupled by using two different laser sources, materials for thermal imaging and thermal ablation. In the case of diagnostic applications, nanothermometers are used for monitoring ischemia and inflammation in vivo [36]. As can be noted, this section encompassed reports that facilitated cancer diagnosis only in cells and not in tissue samples. One of the possible reasons for limited studies involving tissue samples could be the attenuation of the fluorescing light by a large number of cells in the considered tissue sample [20].

7.3 Vibrational Spectroscopy-Based Detection Strategies

Rotational, vibrational and electronic energies of a molecule increase when it absorbs EM radiation. Upon interaction of the molecule with the incident EM wave, a transition occurs from the ground state to an excited state. The three energy levels could be ordered in the following way based on their energies: rotational $<$ vibrational $<$ electronic. Transitions in the vibrational energy levels are modulated by IR radiation. In a harmonic diatomic oscillator model, interaction with EM waves mediates changes in internuclear distances between the vibrating masses m and M. The vibrational frequency (ν) is characteristic of the structure of the molecule under investigation and depends on the reduced mass of the oscillator and strength of the bond between m and M (Eq. 7.1). However, in the case of large amplitudes of vibration, aspects of repulsive forces between vibrating atoms and their dissociation should be considered, which are modelled by anharmonic oscillators [37].

$$\nu = \frac{1}{2\pi} \cdot \sqrt{\frac{\mathrm{f}}{\mu}} \tag{7.1}$$

$$\mu - \frac{mM}{m + M} \tag{7.2}$$

This section encompasses a brief description of two kinds of vibrational spectroscopy, IR and Raman spectroscopy and their use in the diagnosis of cervical cancer.

7.3.1 Infrared Spectroscopy-Based Detection

For molecules to be IR active, their dipole moment should vary with vibrations. The dipole moment of a molecule represents the product of charge difference and distance between two charge centres. As the molecule vibrates, there will be fluctuations in electron densities around the atoms and this may change the dipole moment associated with it. These charge fluctuations generate an electric field that, when interacting with EM radiation, tends to absorb those with the same frequency as the molecules' natural vibrational frequency, resulting in an increase in vibrational amplitude. For molecules possessing a permanent dipole moment, the electron cloud will be amassed around the electronegative atom. Subsequently, the fluctuations in electron density will cause significant variations in dipole moment; hence such molecules are IR active [37].

IR spectroscopy, a very sensitive technique, is popularly used for identification and structural analysis of a variety of organic and inorganic compounds. The obtained absorption/transmission spectrum is characteristic of the molecule under investigation. According to the Boltzmann distribution, many of the molecules occupy the ground state ($n = 0$) and excitation to the next higher energy level ($n = 1$) is more prominent. Such excitations are referred to as allowed or fundamental transitions. Further, the majority of chemical functionalities are absorbed in these wavenumber regions of 4000–400 cm^{-1} [37]. The initial IR instruments employed a dispersive element such as a prism or grating to separate individual frequency components emitted from the IR source. However, these dispersive IR instruments can only perform slow scanning. Hence, in order to increase the speed and facilitate simultaneous scanning of all frequencies, the Fourier transform infrared (FTIR) instrument was developed. FTIR consists of a source, an interferometer arrangement and a detector. The interferometer is made up of a beam splitter, a stationary flat mirror and a movable flat mirror. After passing through the beam splitter, IR beam produces two optical beams of which one is reflected off from flat immovable mirror, while the other reflects off from mirror which moves a short distance away from the beam splitter. This setup results in interference between two beams and the produced IR beam interacts with the sample. The interferogram is decoded by Fourier transformation and a plot of intensity vs frequency is obtained [38].

Although genomic studies have gained immense recognition for cancer diagnosis, tumours display extended heterogeneity, limiting their cell level characterisation ability [39]. Histological analysis only gives qualitative information pertaining to cell morphology, size and stain variations. In this regard, IR spectroscopy, which can provide quantitative information about biomolecules such as lipids, proteins, carbohydrates and nucleic acid, proves to be a fitting contender for biological sample analysis. Further, the changes associated with tissue biochemistry such as lipid peroxidation, protein aggregation and more which precede or are manifested by the disease are reflected in the IR spectrum, which can indeed be used to probe the various stages associated with the transition from normal to cancerous tissue [40]. Owing to this technique's relevance in cancer diagnosis, this section encompasses some works pertaining to the use of IR spectroscopy towards cervical cancer diagnosis.

Mordechai et al. [41] carried out FTIR analysis on formalin fixed biopsy samples and highlighted the differences in IR spectrum associated with cervical cancer and melanoma tissue samples. It was seen that cervical cancerous tissue samples had lower absorption in the wavenumber region of 900–1185 cm^{-1}. This region corresponds to glycogen groups, which are associated with cell maturation and may decrease with the differentiation of normal cells into neoplastic cells [42]. Further, with an altered metabolism and increased cell replication characteristics, there is a corresponding increase in the transcription of cancer cells. This is reflected as increase in intensity of anti-symmetric phosphate peaks of DNA and RNA, occurring between 1185–1300 cm^{-1}. Combined utilisation of peak ratios for RNA (1121 cm^{-1})/DNA (1020 cm^{-1}) and glycogen/asymmetric phosphate content was reported to be a reliable strategy for detection of cervical cancer [41].

Ethanol preserves the architecture of cell organelles and facilitates rapid dehydration of cellular material, thereby avoiding the adsorption of any trace molecule. Also, ethanol preserves samples by avoiding staining or fixing procedures. Cervical spatulas and brushes can be preserved in an absolute ethanol solution. Hence, Wood et al. [43] performed IR analysis on ethanol preserved samples in a multicavity IR cell. The cell being single crystalline minimised the fringing effects, removed water from samples and further facilitated their effective spreading, which enabled easy identification of contaminants. FTIR spectra were obtained for normal epithelial cells and cervical cancer cells. Bands corresponding to glycogen and symmetric modes of phosphates were observed to be largely suppressed in the cervical cancer cells. Further, intense peaks corresponding to anti-symmetric phosphate bands were obtained. Depending on the characteristic differences in the spectra, they were classified as type 1 and type 2. A multivariate statistical method of principal component analysis (PCA) was incorporated in the study and appropriately tailored to aid the analysis for cytologists. Subsequently, abnormal and normal cervical cells were appropriately classified and the work highlighted the potential for spectroscopy of biological samples coupled with computational analysis to aid in the diagnosis of cervical cancer [43].

Synchrotron sources produce EM radiation due to the tangential movement of electrons in a circular unit and are further accelerated by magnetic fields. They could act as smaller sized excitation sources and contribute to minimal thermal noise during analysis. Thus, these sources could be potentially used for IR spectroscopy analysis. Hence, Faolain et al. [44] carried out IR analysis using a synchrotron source. The group performed analysis on dewaxed fixed samples and unfixed frozen samples and compared their corresponding spectra. In the case of dewaxed fixed samples, characteristic peaks were seen for glycogen and symmetric phosphate groups in normal epithelial and basal cells. In the case of connective tissue samples, amide peaks from proteins were obtained. However, in the case of invasive carcinoma cells, significant absorption bands corresponding to nucleic acid were not obtained. Analysis of frozen, unfixed tissue samples revealed significant intensity changes for all epithelial, basal cells and connective tissue. Nucleic acid peaks were reported to be more prominent for basal cells. Furthermore, splitting of amide peaks was observed in the case of connective tissue samples. Although analysis of frozen samples pertaining to invasive carcinoma was not performed in this work, the authors highlighted the enhanced nucleic acid peaks associated with basal cells and envisaged similar spectrum characteristics for cervical carcinoma cells owing to the cancerous origination from basal cells [44].

Although IR spectroscopy offers advantages such as being non-destructive, highly sensitive and requiring only small sample volumes for analysis, it has certain disadvantages. The major disadvantage is interference from water, which overlaps with many proteins found in biological samples, making information on the latter inconspicuous. Albeit in vitro studies involving ethanol preserved samples can do away with this interference, it is not possible to utilise this technique in vivo, thus necessitating conventional biopsy or other minimally invasive procedures for cancer diagnosis. Further, blood and cellular debris commonly associated with the cervix have been reported to affect IR analysis. Also, IR spectra of tissue samples subjected to formalin fixation and paraffinisation experience interference due to fixing reagents [44]. In this regard, deparaffinisation of samples ought to be carried out prior to IR analysis. In addition, processing of spectrum images followed by computational analysis may give away unique and varying features associated with samples, which could be harnessed for diagnostic purposes [43].

7.3.2 Raman Spectroscopy-Based Detection

An EM wave, on interacting with a material undergoes a shift in its wavelength which may be attributed to material absorption or reflection or scattering. Raman spectroscopy involves analysis of scattered EM waves. Phonons, the quantised form of molecules' vibrations, interact with the incoming photons from the incident monochromatic laser beam. On interacting with incoming photons, phonons from the ground state are excited to higher energy levels, become unstable and thus emit photons of the same frequency. This is known as elastic or Rayleigh scattering and occurs at about 99% per incident EM wave. Further, the emitted photons do not give any information about the molecule. Conversely, inelastic or Raman scattering results in changes in energy in the emitted photons. For instance, phonons may absorb energy from incoming photons and shift to energy levels just above the ground state and thus emit photons of low energy, resulting in a Stokes shift. Otherwise, the incoming photons may be excited by phonons and thus the emitted EM wave may be of higher frequency, resulting in an anti-Stokes shift. The latter is much rarer, hence less intense, and thus much of Raman scattering involves contribution from Stokes shift. Thus, notch filters, tuneable filters and others are used to selectively remove the Rayleigh component from the scattered waves and enhance the quality of Raman spectra. The wavelength of emitted photons, which are either low or high in comparison to the incident photons, is characteristic of the vibrational energy of the molecule. Further, the polarisability of a vibrating molecule is frequency dependent, so changes in polarisation of a molecule in interaction with an incident EM wave provides useful information about its composition [45]. Unlike IR spectroscopy, interference signals from water molecules are suppressed in Raman spectroscopy because different selection rules apply to Raman and IR. This renders Raman highly meritorious for biological sample analysis. [44].

The greater spatial and spectral resolution associated with Raman spectroscopy confers its greater sensitivity over IR analysis. This was evident from the work carried out by Faolain et al. [44]. In their study, they observed that normal epithelial cells exhibited glycogen bands whereas carcinoma cells showed enhanced peaks for DNA owing to increased replication activity in cancer cells [44]. The above work could be considered as the first generation utility of Raman analysis for cervical cancer detection. Researchers, over the last few decades, have focused on building research grade micro-Raman instruments to facilitate analysis of single cells that could screen for cancer cells and even detect bacteria or viruses. However, parameters such as the wavelength of the irradiation source and the substrate housing need to be optimized and judiciously chosen, respectively. For instance, green laser excitation elicits strong autofluorescence in biological media and hence the NIR irradiation source is preferred. Further, trace amounts of rare-earth metals present in glass substrates produce fluorescence bands, obscuring the Raman spectra of the biological samples. Considering these factors, Kamemoto et al. [46] performed Raman analysis (at 785 nm) on frozen slices of cervical tissue samples mounted on aluminium metal coated glass substrate. Apart from eliciting fewer background signals in Raman analysis, the aluminium coated glass substrate enhanced the contrast for microscopic imaging and also enhanced the Raman bands associated with samples. The absence of peaks at 854 cm^{-1} and 938 cm^{-1} indicating a dip in collagen and elastin content along with fewer broader bands for C-H vibrations were reported as characteristic Raman features of cancerous cervical tissues [46].

Raman analysis has been used for in vivo detection of cervical cancer, owing to minimized interference from water molecules [42]. Optical fibres, in this regard, have been tried for in vivo Raman analysis. However, as these fibres contain silica, they produce strong Raman peaks that interfere with the spectrum of cervical cancer tissues [46]. Also, owing to the low Raman cross-section associated with biological samples, laser source of greater power may be required to produce spectra with conspicuous peaks, which could potentially elevate the problems associated with unintended heating of biological tissues [46]. Hence, apart from optimising spectra processing to identify characteristic differences between cervical cancer afflicted samples and normal samples, the pre-mentioned aspects pertaining to laser irradiation medium and source wavelength must be optimised so that Raman can plausibly be translated for in vivo cancer diagnosis applications.

7.4 FET Based Sensors

The previous chapters encompassed reports of different types of electrical sensors such as voltammetric, amperometric and impedimetric sensors for cervical cancer detection. This section includes a discussion of field effect transistor (FET) based sensors for the diagnosis of cervical cancer. FET offers several advantages over bipolar junction transistor (BJT) such as low thermal noise, higher gain to drain resistance, low-power switching and effective miniaturisation [47].

BioFETs consist of biological recognition elements attached to the gate regions, where the underlying channel acts as a transducer and produces a signal corresponding to the changes in analyte concentration. Voltage applied across the gate electrodes will promote the charges present in the electrolyte solution in the channel to move in a direction perpendicular to its flow and hence vary the interfacial potential across the gate electrode. This in-turn influences the channel resistance, whose values are characteristics of the composition of the surface of the gate electrode [48]. Attachment of biomolecules to the gate electrode surface can be achieved by simple physical adsorption, sol-gel process, Langmuir Blodgett (LB) film deposition, cross-linking, covalent attachment or gel entrapment procedures [49–52]. Albeit physical adsorption is a simple immobilisation strategy, the possibility for desorption of recognition element exists. The LB film method results in porous or defective surface layer formation and hence has to be performed under optimum pressure conditions. Crosslinkers are multifunctional reagents and thus may facilitate interaction between biomolecules and components of a polymer or gel matrix. Covalent attachment is a highly reliable immobilisation strategy for biomolecules, which involves the formation of stable chemical bonds with the gate electrode surface. BioFETs may be broadly classified as catalytic and affinity-based. Catalytic BioFETs are made by immobilising biocatalysts like enzymes on gate electrodes, which interact with a specific substrate or product. These changes in the concentration of enzymes or products influence the current flow through the channel and the corresponding analyte concentrations can be obtained. Affinity-based BioFETs involve immobilisation of antibodies, DNA or receptor like biomolecules which bind irreversibly to their corresponding target molecules without the aid of any enzyme or other biocatalysts. They are further categorised as label-free and labeled affinity BioFETs. In the case of label-free affinity immuno-BioFETs, which involve interaction between antigen and antibodies, the changes in charge distribution owing to the formation of antigen-antibody complex are reflected in drain current values and hence antigen concentrations can be obtained. Similarly, in the case of ss-DNA modified BioFETs, the hybridisation with the complementary DNA strand results in charge distribution changes and the corresponding changes in drain current values are indicative of the target DNA concentration. Labelled BioFETs majorly utilise enzyme labelled antibodies or receptor molecules, where interaction of enzyme with deliberately added substrates yields products or reduces label concentration, which in-turn provide information about the analyte molecules present in the sample [53].

Carbon nanotube-based FET (CNTFET) offers high conductivity owing to its material properties. Furthermore, with changes in the diameter of the CNTs, corresponding variations in the threshold voltage could be observed. Hence, Gopinath et al. [54] utilised a CNTFET-based nano-biosensor for the detection of cervical cancer. The current flow across the CNT channel is modulated by voltage applied across two gate electrodes. When antigen-containing analyte samples are placed on a biosensor array, they spread and interact with the antibodies present on each biosensor in the array. Subsequently, significant amounts of analyte will be available in the vicinity of the added region (referred to as the core) and lesser amounts of analyte will tend to reach the periphery of the biosensor array. As a result, electro-potentials generated by analyte interaction with the biosensor will be lower in the periphery than in the core. In order to render electro-potential contributions from periphery equally significant, the group set pre-defined voltage values of 0 V, 0.2 V and 0.4 V for the core, middle and periphery biosensor array regions, respectively. The resultant current output is converted to voltage via a current to voltage converter and fed to differential amplifier, where a pre-defined voltage obtained for non-cancer samples is set as the reference. The top gate on CNTFET was modified with a cervical specific antibody (CSA) and the back gate was set with a pre-defined bias voltage obtained from the reference circuit utilised in the work. The load voltage obtained due to drain current passing through a load resistor was indicative of analyte concentration in the sample. This setup significantly improved the sensitivity of the sensor and proved to be suitable for biosensor applications [54].

Recently, reduced graphene oxide-based FET (rGO-FET) biosensors have gained attention towards a variety of diagnostically relevant bioassays, ranging from detection of Ebola glycoproteins [55] to SARS-CoV-2 spike protein detection [56]. Aspermair et al. [57] fabricated the rGO-FET biosensor for HPV-16 E7 protein detection. The work involved functionalising the glass surfaces in the interdigitated electrodes with 3-amino-propyltriethoxysilane (APTES) and modifying the electrode surface with rGO, by initialising GO deposition and reducing it with hydrazine. The modified electrode was immersed in pyrene carboxylic acid and pyrene polyethylene glycol mixture, and to the EDC/NHS activated acid groups, E7 protein specific aptamer sequences were attached. Electrode surface modifications were confirmed via XPS studies. Real-time recombinant HPV-16 E6 protein binding with an aptamer modified rGO-FET biosensor revealed corresponding changes in current values with a Langmuir isotherm based binding curve pattern. Analysis performed using insulin, which is of similar size to that of HPV-16 E6 protein, revealed the sensor to exhibit little changes in current values. It was reasoned that owing to insulin's negative charge, the effect of applied electric field is counteracted, whereas this was not the case with HPV-16 E6 protein aptamers and hence significant current changes could be seen. The sensor exhibited similar performance and sensitivity characteristics on both PBS containing HPV-16 E6 protein and spiked saliva samples. The limit of detection for the sensor was reported to be 1.75 nM and it exhibited long-term stability [57].

Low-cost fabrication and the requirement of minimal sample for analysis are some of the distinct advantages of BioFETs. Further, with necessary processing, differentially expressed and disease relevant analytes present in serum or saliva samples can be analysed using FET based sensors [57]. This circumvents the laborious and invasive procedures of biopsy, tissue fixation and further opens up the arena of non-invasive diagnosis. However, the electro-potential changes due to the formation of antigen-antibody complexes or DNA duplexes in the case of label-free immune-BioFETs and DNA BioFETs are not significantly discernible, thereby necessitating the use of labels such as enzymes. Because of this, certain reports suggest the utilisation of techniques such as electron impedance spectroscopy to comment on antigen–antibody complex formation. However, aspects of FET passivation, biomolecule immobilisation on the gate electrode surface, and channel size and shape are important parameters that must be optimised in order to obtain drain current values that correspond to the analyte concentration in samples.

7.5 Mechanical Biosensors

Advancements in the technologies of micro- and nano-fabrication have paved the way for the development of mechanical sensors with nano-sized moving parts. These sensors capitalise on their idiosyncratic properties such as providing a pronounced mass resolution, where the total mass of the fabricated device is proportional to the added mass that needs to be detected [58]. Secondly, mechanical compliance sharply increases with scale reduction. In other words, the ability of the sensor to undergo displacement or deformation increases with decreasing scales of dimensions, from bulk to micro/nano-dimensions. This results in the amplification of force response, opening up avenues for measurement of diminutive forces governing biological systems. Thirdly, such mechanical sensors exhibit fast response times [59].

With these merits, mechanical biosensors could be distinguished into four kinds based on the chemical interactions happening between the biosensor and the analyte [59]. These are:

(a) Affinity-based: Affinity between the target molecule and functionalised component(s) at the device surface is utilised to achieve increased target recognition and capturing.
(b) Fingerprint: Multiple functionalised layers which exhibit unique binding affinities towards analytes are present in the sensor ensemble and this arrangement is employed for the identification of the target molecules.
(c) Separation-based: Spatio-temporal delineation of flowing target molecules and immobilised components on the sensor surface results in a differential chemical affinity pattern.
(d) Spectrometric: Mass or optical properties of the target are utilised to aid in its sensing.

In addition, based on the physical processes that govern the operation of mechanical biosensors, they could be grouped into surface stress and dynamic mode sensors. The first type of sensor measures the quasistatic deflection of a microscopic cantilever caused by the binding of target molecules to the functional groups on the sensor surface. As a result of such a binding process, a surface stress is developed due to electrostatic attraction/repulsion, steric effects, hydration or entropic interactions. The deflection caused is measured using a setup that involves a laser beam reflecting off the cantilever. Specifically, in the cases of proteins and DNA, piezoelectric readouts have been employed [59]. In the case of dynamic mode sensors, they oscillate at their characteristic resonance frequency in the absence of target molecules. In their presence, this characteristic frequency shifts, proportional to the number of molecules landing on the cantilever [60].

Predominantly, in several studies involving the detection of cervical cancer biomarkers, the affinity-based and spectrometric kinds of mechanical biosensors have been employed owing to their simplicity and high sensitivity. However, high affinity mechanical biosensors that rely heavily on the affinity between the target molecule and the functionalised component, are typically found only in the liquid phase. Hence, post the target capture, the detection of the target has to be performed in situ, which would be strongly affected by viscous damping, thereby reducing the mass resolution expected out of mechanical biosensors [59].

In this context, the spectrometric kinds of mechanical biosensors have gained much attention and traction amongst researchers, owing to their simple design resulting in low instrumentation costs, prospective real-time detection, possibility of label-free detection and high sensitivity [59]. One such category of mechanical biosensors is the quartz-crystal microbalances (QCM).

QCM-based biosensing employs mechanical resonators in the dimensional range of centimetres, which are capable of measuring the inertial mass and its corresponding changes in the target moiety(ies), amassing on their surfaces [61]. Commonly, this microbalance utilises a base of a thin disk of AT-cut quartz sided by electrodes on either side [62]. Before the landing of these moieties, the resonators vibrate at their characteristic resonant frequency. Upon amassment of the target molecules, a significant shift in that resonant frequency occurs and is subsequently tracked in real-time by electronic means [61, 62]. This relationship between frequency and mass is given by the Sauerbrey equation:

$$\Delta f = -\frac{2f_0^2}{A\sqrt{\rho_q \mu_q}}\Delta m \tag{7.3}$$

where f_0 is the resonant frequency in Hz, Δf is the normalised frequency change in Hz, Δm is the mass change due to the amassment of the target molecules in grams (g), A is the piezoelectrically active area or the area between the electrodes in cm^2, ρ_q is the quartz density equal to 2.648 g/cm^3 and μ_q is the shear modulus of quartz for the AT-cut crystal equal to 2.947×10^{11} g cm^{-1} s^{-2} [62].

It is to be noted that the above Sauerbrey equation is applicable under conditions where the amassed mass over the sensor surface must be rigid; the distribution of the amassed mass must be even over the surface of the sensor and the frequency change is less than 5%. If the frequency change exceeds this limit of 5%, then the Z-match method ought to be used for determination of the mass of the target [63].

Since most of the biological detection involves liquid samples, the Sauerbrey equation stands limited in its application to determine masses in such samples. Kanazawa et al. proposed a modified form of the Sauerbrey equation, taking into account the decrease in the resonant frequency as a result of the liquid viscosity [64]. Mathematically, the modified equation was given by.

$$\Delta f = f_0^{3/2}\sqrt{\frac{\eta_l \rho_l}{\pi \rho_q \mu_q n}}\Delta m \tag{7.4}$$

where ρ_l is the liquid density, η_l is the liquid viscosity and n is the mode number [64].

With this background on mechanical and especially piezoelectric biosensors based on QCMs, discussion on the application of such sensors for the detection of cervical cancer would be essential. Meritoriously, these sensors are preferred owing to their label-free detection and swift monitoring of DNA hybridisation predominantly. Considering these merits, a collaborative study performed by Atti et al. involved a hybrid method with PCR and QCM for specific and sensitive detection of HPV, in 2007 [65]. They employed an ensemble of probes that were specific and degenerate for detecting and genotyping the HPV in human specimens. Three piezoelectric biosensors were developed that involved a degenerate probe for detection of various HPV strains like HPV-6, 11, 16, 18, 33 and highly specific probes for the high-risk HPV types, HPV 16 and 18. The methodology of this study involved an innovative strategy wherein a degenerate biosensor was initially developed, which had the ability to identify qualitatively the presence/absence of the target HPV virus in the considered sample, without genotype identification. They were able to design a 31-mer oligonucleotide probe comprising the conserved 11-mer sequence across HPV strains (HPV-16, 33, 18, 6 and 11) and an extended 20-mer region with 4 degenerate points. The significance of these degenerate points is that the different HPV strains differentiate themselves at these points. Furthermore, if this HPV degenerate sensor furnished samples that were positive for HPV, they were then considered to be detected using the HPV-16 or HPV-18 specific biosensors. The immobilised probes on these specific biosensors were rationally chosen, in view of the fact that the region of the HPV genome that was conserved the least corresponded to the differentiator between HPV-16 and 18 genotypes. All the probes in this study were immobilised with the help of a biotin–streptavidin pair. PCR was used as the amplification method required for increasing the DNA content before allowing the sample to come in contact with the modified QCM surface consisting of the immobilised probes. The authors, in this study, have claimed that their technique of using degenerate and specific probes could be extended for the detection of other microorganisms that are difficult to detect due to their high mutation rates [65].

Furthermore, a research group from Thailand developed a hybrid detection technique, but it involves QCM and loop-mediated isothermal amplification (LAMP) [66]. This LAMP technique of amplifying DNA was first reported by a collaborative research study in Japan in 2000 [67]. LAMP stands unique as an amplification technique because of its enhanced specificity and efficiency along with the merit of serving as a rapid technique (less than an hour required for amplification) under isothermal conditions. In this method, a DNA polymerase and four specifically designed primers capable of identifying six unique sequences present in the target DNA are utilised. Quoting the procedure from the report itself, which goes: "*An inner primer containing sequences of the sense and anti-sense strands of target DNA initiates LAMP. The ensuing strand displacement DNA synthesis primed by an outer primer releases a single-stranded DNA. This serves as a template for DNA synthesis primed by the second inner and outer primers that hybridise with the other end of the target, producing a stem-loop DNA structure. In subsequent cycles, one inner primer hybridises to the loop on the product and initiates displacement DNA synthesis, yielding the original stem-loop DNA and a new stem-loop DNA with a stem twice as long*" [67]. The mechanism of this amplification technique is shown in Fig. 7.2.

Earlier, the same group had reported the qualitative detection of HPV-58 viral DNA using this methodology. However, in the chosen study, they have reported the application of this hybrid detection technique for HPV-16 viral DNA in 31 cervical cancer tissues that were considered. Using TaqMan-quantitative PCR, the viral copy number of HPV-16 DNA was identified by amplifying the E6 region using the TaqMan probe, acting as the control method. In parallel, the QCM system that was

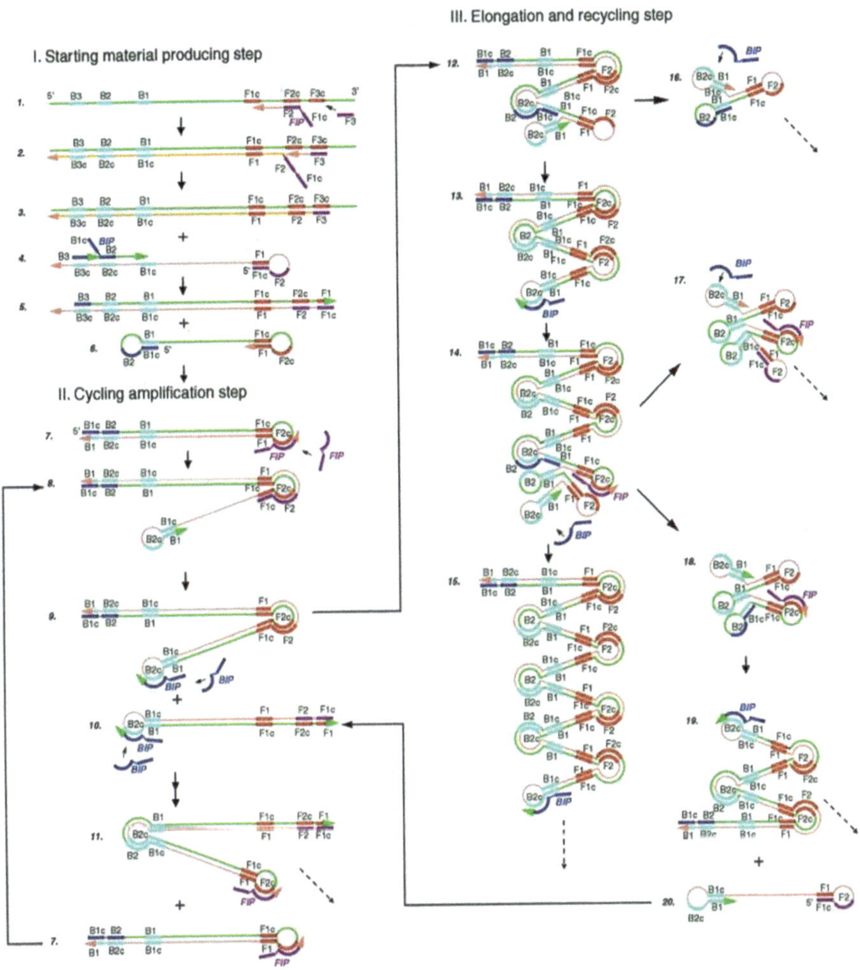

Fig. 7.2 Schematic representation of LAMP mechanism [67]

used for this study comprised a QCM chamber along with a heating box requisite for maintenance of isothermal conditions for LAMP reactions. The QCM system was modified by a thiol-self-assembly procedure followed by immobilisation of avidin, whereas the amplified products were biotinylated. The authors claimed that the LAMP-QCM method exhibited a ten-fold higher sensitivity method along with a quicker analysis time (30 mins) against the TaqMan-qPCR control method (3 h) [66].

Apart from the predominantly considered mechanical biosensor methodology in the form of QCM, there are interests in the development of surface acoustic wave (SAW) biosensors for the detection of cervical cancer. Generally, SAW devices work by generating and detecting acoustic waves with the help of interdigital transducers (IDT) present on a piezoelectric crystal surface [68]. Consequently, acoustic energy gets increasingly confined to the surface of the crystal in the acoustic wavelength range, irrespective of substrate thickness. This behaviour makes these devices highly sensitive to any surface changes like mass and viscosity changes, predominantly [69]. SAW devices were first reported as a sensor by Wohltjen and Dessy employing Rayleigh-type SAWs, where the device was coated with a polymer layer sensitive to an organic gas [70]. Later, these SAW devices evolved into biosensing with initial challenges as the SAW devices designed for gas sensing suffered from pronounced attenuation owing to displacements occurring perpendicular to the sensor surface when immersed in aqueous samples. Such displacements result in the radiation of compression waves, termed as leaky waves into the aqueous medium, causing unwanted attenuation [71].

Although leaky waves are considered undesirable, a novel biosensor based on these leaky waves (LSAW) has been developed for the detection of cervical cancer. In this study, a peptide nucleic acid (PNA) probe was used against the conventional use of DNA probes for HPV in cervical cancer detection owing to mismatched hybridisation between non-target sequences and DNA sequences and lower detection sensitivity due to smaller DNA probes. PNA, advantageously, consists of a synthetic peptide backbone (instead of the natural sugar phosphate backbone in nucleic acids) that is achiral and uncharged. This qualifies PNA to bind to homopurine targets in double-stranded DNA through a strand displacement mechanism, against the triple helix formation conventionally observed in the case of natural oligonucleotides. The PNA–DNA complex remains stable when the Watson-Crick base pairing PNA strand is present in the anti-parallel orientation to the DNA strand and the Hoogsteen strand is present in the parallel orientation to the DNA strand [72].

Furthermore, the LSAW device used for this study was comprised of double two-port resonators that included a detection channel along with a reference channel, which was operated at a high frequency of 100 MHz. Subsequently, the gold surface of the LSAW device was modified to immobilise the PNA probes using the thiol self-assembly method [72]. In summary, this group developed a LSAW biosensor employing a bis-PNA probe which allows for direct detection of HPV without the need for PCR, where the PNA probe was highly specific towards HPV-18 but not HPV-16 with a sensitivity seven times greater than that of a QCM sensor [72].

Mechanical biosensors have evolved, both horizontally and vertically. In other words, a lot of new kinds of mechanical biosensors have been developed (horizontal evolution) as well as novel modifications of a given method (vertical evolution). In this context, apart from QCM and SAW biosensors, microelectromechanical system (MEMS) based biosensors for cervical cancer detection have been reported. One such study involved the development of an on-chip antibody-based detection method for cervical cancer utilising a MEMS device for recognition and capture of cervical cancer cells using α_6 integrin receptors. It is very well known clinically that the increased expression of $\alpha_6\beta_4$ integrin at the injury site leads to HPV infection. A microfluidic platform was fabricated from polydimethylsiloxane (PDMS) elastomer, followed by the conventional channel fabrication method. The PDMS surface was subsequently modified using 3-mercaptopropyltrimethosilane (MTS) and N-γ-

maleimidobutyryloxy succinimide ester (GMBS) solutions. Later, dilute amounts of the antibody solution were passed through the modified channels for immobilisation. It was mainly observed in this study that longer channels in the MEMS platform could result in higher sensitivity to capturing target cervical cancer cells on the PDMS surface [73].

The field of developing mechanical biosensors for cervical cancer detection is still an open arena considering the challenges from developing better capture agents or probes to integrating ensembles of nano-sensors with the help of conventional microfabrication techniques. The road ahead in this arena will be the design and development of mechanical biosensors that are capable of high-throughput studies at the scale of individual cells and molecules.

7.6 PCR Biosensors

Notwithstanding the burgeoning methods of detection reported and developed for cervical cancer, PCR remains idiosyncratic owing to its ability to precisely detect the mutated strains of HPV induced cervical carcinoma. This is because compared to its fellow DNA viruses, HPV cannot be detected by conventional cell culture methods. With the extensive reports and literature on specific changes in the L1 and E6 regions of the HPV genome, variegated PCR or hybridisation-based methodologies have been devised. Furthermore, there are at present several HPV kits that have been FDA-approved, like the Hybrid Capture II, Cervista™ HPV HR and Cobas® HPV Test for detection of high-risk HPV in DNA samples isolated from cervical cancer patients [74]. This background clearly indicates the significance of using PCR for specific detection of HPV induced cervical cancer, setting the basis for discussion on various developments in this direction.

Prakash et al., in one such novel study, reported the usage of nested multiplex PCR (NMPCR) for detection of mucosal HPVs, initially followed by simultaneous typing of HPV-16 and HPV-18 from cervical carcinoma and cervical intraepithelial neoplasia samples [74]. Multiplex PCR was proposed as a modified PCR technique to address the shortcomings of uniplex/conventional PCR, which were inadequate test sample volume and low diagnostic capacity. Hence, in this modified technique, various target sequences could be amplified by the inclusion of a corresponding number of pairs of primers in the chain reaction. Such a development in PCR comes against the conventional focus on optimising the factors influencing annealing and extension rates, like annealing temperature, poor design of primers, and enzyme activity, predominantly [75]. Hence, NMPCR was just an incremental development wherein multiple rounds of multiplex PCR were carried out. In this study, they were able to obtain a sensitivity at the picogram level for the detection of HPV-specific gene sequence and the specificity to detect the HPV-16 sequence [74].

Even though PCR is credited with high clinical specificity and sensitivity, it is often limited to being used in population-scale screening under low resource conditions, owing to its high price. A study carried out by Surriabre et al. provides a reprieve from this shortcoming by proposing a low-cost PCR method involving the combined use of PCR with BSGP 5+/6+ primers and PCR with pU primers. To compare the efficacy of their methodology, the HC2 system developed by Qiagen was used as the control, which could identify 13 HPV genotypes (16, 18, 31, 33, 35, 39, 45, 51, 52, 56, 58, 59 and 68). The BSGP primers consist of 9 forward primers and 3 reverse primers. Kappa values indicating the degree of agreement between the techniques were calculated for each of the individual PCR methods (BSGP and pU separately) and their combination. From their analysis, it was found that the kappa value for the combined technique (0.82) was in agreement with the commercial control HC2 system and higher when the methods were considered separately. Furthermore, the combined technique has a greater sensitivity (88.7%) against the individual methods (BSGP – 77.4% and pU – 60.9%) along with a comparable specificity of 95.1% against BSGP's 96.9% and pU's 96.5% when performed independently [76].

Furthermore, coupling the advantages of PCR such as the ability to perform the analysis with a very low sample volume, the capability to verify the presence of multiple infections and precise determination of genotype, along with the increased sensitivity associated with the fluorescence method, has been reported by Kim et al. [77].

In the reported study, the group developed a DNA chip which is comprised of an ensemble solution that has the amplified DNA products produced by biotinylated GP primers from PCR along with a fluorescently active streptavidin solution. In this setup, when the patient's sample is loaded onto the chip, in the presence of HPV 16 or 18, they observed a fluorescence signal from the corresponding HPV type DNA chip only. They claimed that the sensitivity of this combined assay was much greater than an individual PCR run to detect the HPV types along with a significant reduction in the response time from about 4 h for PCR to 30 mins for this combined system [77].

Similar to the above study, but in a different setup altogether, the lateral flow assay was adjoined with PCR for endeavouring high sensitivity and multiplex detection, as shown in Fig. 7.3. The bottom line of their detection strategy is the following: fluorescently labelled detection probes were used in the PCR. Subsequently, when these PCR products are added to the lateral flow strip which already comprises the immobilised capture probes, due to capillary movement, three elements such as the detection probe, the capture probe, and the single-stranded PCR product will form a sandwich-like product on hybridisation with each other. This would then be detected by using a fluorescent reader. This group restricted themselves for the detection of four common HPV types, namely HPV 6, 11, 16, and 18. They also added an internal positive control in the form of the human β-globin gene, so as to prevent false negatives. Multiplex PCR was employed wherein the five targets were amplified in a single reaction using GP primers for the four HPV types and a separate primer pair for the internal control. Linear-after-the-exponential (LATE) PCR was employed for this study so that they could obtain abundant single-stranded PCR products for the hybridisation process [78].

LATE-PCR refers to an asymmetric method wherein primers are thoughtfully designed for unequal concentrations in such a way that the melting temperature of the limiting primer is at least greater than the melting temperature of the excess

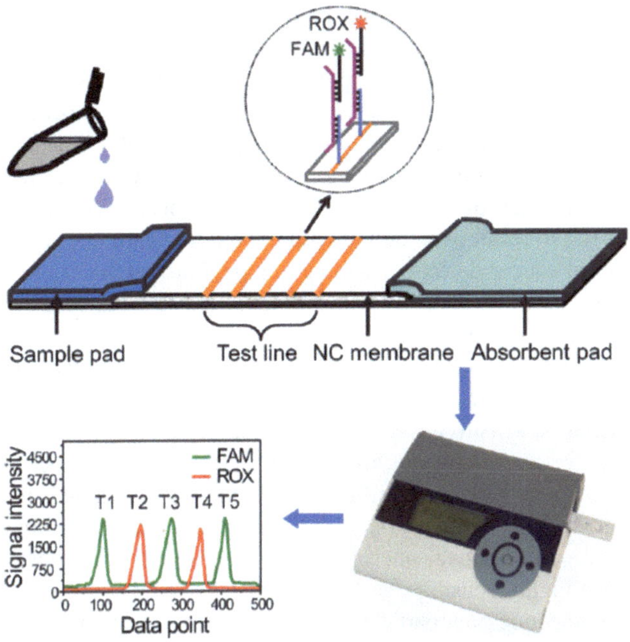

Fig. 7.3 Schematic illustration of configuration and measurement principle of fluorescent probe-based nucleic acid lateral flow assay (Reprinted (adapted) with permission from [78], Copyright (2014) American Chemical Society)

primer. This method is characterised by an initial exponential phase wherein the efficiency of amplification is the same as that of symmetric PCR and a later linear phase wherein the single-stranded product is generated for additional cycles as soon as the limiting primer is depleted in the reaction mixture [79].

Subsequently, in their procedure, one pair of detection and capture probes was ascribed to each of their four HPV targets where the capture probe was modified with a 3′ poly(dT) spacer for ensuring high binding efficiency post immobilisation. This was followed by biotinylation of the capture probe and subsequent mixing with neutravidin so that the capture probe could be immobilised on the nitrocellulose membrane. The study claimed several merits, such as a lower response time of just 30 min (similar to the previous study), ease of methodology compared to conventionally used post-PCR analysis like Southern blot techniques, and mainly, a high-throughput multiplex lateral flow assay system capable of acting as a point of care testing device [78].

7.7 Other Optical Biosensors

Optical biosensors, by far, are the most conspicuously tapped kind of biosensors in the literature owing to their unique optical signal characteristics, like higher sensitivity, immunity to disturbances from external sources and hence, their high stability and low noise, in comparison with other physical signal-based biosensors. Similar to mechanical biosensors, optical biosensors can be easily miniaturised and are capable of chip integration [80]. Generally, optical biosensors are classified into catalytic biosensors and affinity biosensors, where the former employs biocomponents with the ability to recognise the desired biochemical molecule(s) and results in their subsequent conversion into a product(s) by virtue of a chemical reaction. Conversely, the latter kinds of biosensors make use of specific characteristics of the target molecule(s) to result in a binding with the bio-recognition element [81]. With regard to cervical cancer detection, although optical biosensors could be classified into various verticals based on the optical signal chosen, the focus is primed on recently developed novel platforms in this chapter.

Miniaturised bio-chip sensors have gained significant attention as optical biosensors, owing to their merits such as faster completion of on-chip reactions along with increased sensitivity as a result of maintenance of a high concentration gradient across the micro-channel, thereby enhancing mass transport. In addition, biomolecules of interest that are confined within the micro-channels would need to travel a shorter distance by diffusion to reach their reaction sites [82].

In this background, a novel microfluidic microbead array has been reported by Zhang et al. for highly sensitive genotyping of HPV employing a multi-enzyme-labelled oligonucleotide-nanoparticle ensemble as the detection component. They initially fabricated the microfluidic channels using conventional photolithography followed by incubation of these channels with 1% bovine serum albumin (BSA) to prevent non-specific adsorption of microbeads onto the walls of the channels at the time of the introduction of the avidin-functionalised polystyrene microbeads. In parallel, DNA capture probes specific to HPV-16, 18 and 52 types were designed, followed by their functionalisation with biotin. Hence, by biotin-avidin affinity, the DNA probes were attached to the microbeads inside each of the microfluidic channels. In addition, gold nanoparticles were prepared by the conventional chemical method to be conjugated with horseradish peroxidase (HRP) enzyme and thiolated oligonucleotide so that they could be used as labels with the secondary DNA probe; tyramine was biotinylated to act as the substrate for HRP enzyme and electron rich proteins such as casein and BSA were modified chemically by covalent linkage to 4-OH-PPA-NHS (3-(4-hydroxyphenyl) propionic acid *N*-hydroxysuccinimide ester) [83].

In a nutshell, they have developed a methodology wherein the microbeads functionalised with modified electron rich proteins and biotinylated DNA capture probes act as the sensing element, while the gold nanoparticles functionalised with HRP and thiolated oligonucleotide get to detect the genotype of the virus, as shown in Fig. 7.4. Hence, during the detection process, when the desired DNA molecule gets sandwiched between the sensing element and the detecting element, HRP initiates the catalytic oxidation of biotinylated tyramine by hydrogen peroxide to tyramine radicals that have a very short lifetime and are highly reactive. This, in turn, would react with the tyrosine residues and 4-OH-PPA parts of the electron rich proteins in a three-step reaction, resulting in the amassing of multiple biotin molecules on the microbead surface. These molecules could now act as docking

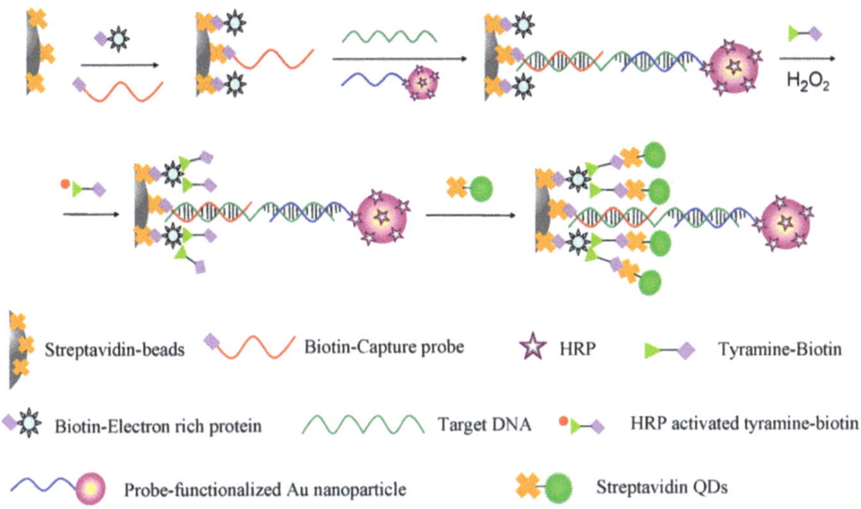

Fig. 7.4 Illustration of microbeads-based multienzyme-nanoparticle amplification for sensitive virus analysis (Copyrights received) [83]

sites for the avidin-conjugated quantum dots (gold nanoparticles) to show fluorescence [83].

The authors have reported that their novel methodology has an absolute detection sensitivity of 10 zeptomoles of target DNA, showing a 1000 fold signal enhancement, ascribed to earlier stated reasons (increased mass transport ability and decreased diffusion distance) [83].

In a similar work, Yue et al. developed a much simpler microfluidic device that used sieved microstructures to form an array of carboxyl-group functionalised microbeads in a single layer allowing for multiplex analysis. In this study, HPV-6, 11, 16 and 18 were chosen for on-chip genotyping. The microbeads were capsulated with two fluorescent dyes with an emission wavelength of 650 and 710 nm. These authors reported a sensitivity of 25 pM of target DNA against zeptomole sensitivity, which could be explained by the trade-off in the number of components used for the study compared to the previous study [84].

In a slightly different strategy, a microarray system employing a bipolar integrated circuit photodiode array (PDA) chip was developed by a group from South Korea. The PDA chip consisted of an array of 8 × 6 photodiodes wherein each photodiode acted as the support for the DNA probe and a 2D photodetector. Here, the p-n junction of each photodiode element was doped with n-type impurities to ensure high leakage current. Subsequently, these photodiode elements were modified by covering them with a very thin layer of silicon dioxide so that the probe DNA could be immobilised on them through organosilane chemistry. In this study, HPV types 16, 18, 56 and 58 were chosen for detection. For the detection strategy, the PDA chips were incubated with anti-biotin antibody conjugated gold nanoparticles, while the target HPV DNA was biotinylated. Upon binding of the above two components, silver precipitates at the surface, blocking the irradiated light (7×6 array of LEDs emitting at 640 nm) and thus, decreasing the photocurrent. This reduction in photocurrent was found to be proportional to the amount of target HPV DNA. This system, as claimed by the authors, exhibited a detection limit of between 1.2 nM and 30 pM based on the silver development time allowed [85].

It is expected that several technical leaps will be made in the future to improve contemporary optical techniques and platforms. One way could be to revise these microfluidic platforms to accommodate smaller reaction chambers so that the processing of nucleic acids, which are currently performed off-chip will be shifted to on-chip and hence improve their clinical utilisation.

7.8 Conclusion

This chapter encompasses various biosensing techniques and detection strategies for cervical cancer detection. It is evident that some of the techniques such as PCR-based detection strategy and vibrational spectroscopy-based diagnosis, require professional personnel to carry out the analysis, thus posing a limitation to their POC translation. Further, one major limitation of the vibrational spectroscopy technique is the requirement of tissue samples, thereby rendering the procedure invasive. In addition, reagents used for tissue fixation methodology interfere with spectroscopy measurements and thus analysis of frozen samples over fixed samples is recommended. Although, QCM possesses high sensitivity, its higher costs limit its extensive usage. In this regard, FET based sensors exhibit greater plausibility for commercial usability. However, aspects of passivation, biomolecule immobilisation and channel geometry must be keenly optimised to ensure reproducible and reliable sensor performance. Although the possibility of intracellular temperature measurements is fascinating, its usability as a cancer diagnosis tool raises issues, since temperature as a sole parameter cannot be used to ascertain the presence of cancer. However, the progress of nanothermometry in vivo shows prospects for the tool's usability in hyperthermia, a widely accepted adjuvant treatment methodology for cancer therapy. In essence, one could get an idea regarding the engineering principles employed and biosensing strategies used and further appreciate the remarkable progress along the lines of cervical cancer diagnosis. However, like many other fields, the field of cervical cancer diagnosis still offers opportunities for further research and devices.

Declaration of Competing Interest The authors declare no conflicts of interest.

Acknowledgements The authors are grateful to the Ministry of Human Resource Development, Government of India for the financial support through *Scheme for Promotion of Academic and Research Collaboration* (*SPARC*) project "SPARC/2018-2019/P402/SL". We also acknowledge the support received from the National Research Foundation (NRF) of Korea for the Basic Science

Research Program funded by the Ministry of Education (NRF-2019R1A6A1A03033215). We are grateful to SASTRA Deemed University, India and SKKU, South Korea for providing infrastructural support.

References

1. Evanko D (2012) A thermometer for cells. Nat Methods 9:328–328. https://doi.org/10.1038/nmeth.1966
2. Karnebogen M, Singer D, Kallerhoff M, Ringert RH (1993) Microcalorimetric investigations on isolated tumorous and non-tumorous tissue samples. Thermochim Acta 229:147–155. https://doi.org/10.1016/0040-6031(93)80322-2
3. Kampinga HH, Dikomey E, Kampinga HH, Dikomey E (2017) Hyperthermic radiosensitization : mode of action and clinical relevance review hyperthermic radiosensitization : mode of action and clinical relevance. Int J Radiat Biol 77:399–408
4. Peer AJ, Grimm MJ, Zynda ER, Repasky EA (2010) Diverse immune mechanisms may contribute to the survival benefit seen in cancer patients receiving hyperthermia. Immunol Res 46:137–154. https://doi.org/10.1007/s12026-009-8115-8
5. Burchardt E, Roszak A (2018) Hyperthermia in cervical cancer – current status. Rep Pract Oncol Radiother 23:595–603. https://doi.org/10.1016/j.rpor.2018.05.006
6. Abadeer NS, Murphy CJ (2016) Recent progress in cancer thermal therapy using gold nanoparticles. J Phys Chem C 120:4691–4716. https://doi.org/10.1021/acs.jpcc.5b11232
7. Thiesen B, Jordan A (2008) Clinical applications of magnetic nanoparticles for hyperthermia. Int J Hyperth 24:467–474. https://doi.org/10.1080/02656730802104757
8. Oyama K, Takabayashi M, Takei Y, Arai S, Takeoka S, Ishiwata S, Suzuki M (2012) Walking nanothermometers: spatiotemporal temperature measurement of transported acidic organelles in single living cells. Lab Chip 12:1591–1593. https://doi.org/10.1039/C2LC00014H
9. Hattori K, Naguro I, Okabe K, Funatsu T, Furutani S, Takeda K, Ichijo H (2016) ASK1 signalling regulates Brown and Beige adipocyte function. Nat Commun 7:11158. https://doi.org/10.1038/ncomms11158
10. Wang D, Huang H, Zhou M, Lu H, Chen J, Chang YT, Gao J, Chai Z, Hu Y (2019) A Thermoresponsive Nanocarrier for mitochondria-targeted drug delivery. Chem Commun 55:4051–4054. https://doi.org/10.1039/c9cc00603f
11. Kucsko G, Maurer PC, Yao NY, Kubo M, Noh HJ, Lo PK, Park H, Lukin MD (2013) Nanometre-scale thermometry in a living cell. Nature 500:54–58. https://doi.org/10.1038/nature12373
12. Zhu X, Feng W, Chang J, Tan Y-W, Li J, Chen M, Sun Y, Li F (2016) Temperature-feedback upconversion nanocomposite for accurate photothermal therapy at facile temperature. Nat Commun 7:10437. https://doi.org/10.1038/ncomms10437
13. Zhu X, Li J, Qiu X, Liu Y, Feng W, Li F (2018) Upconversion nanocomposite for programming combination cancer therapy by precise control of microscopic temperature. Nat Commun 9:2176. https://doi.org/10.1038/s41467-018-04571-4
14. Ferdinandus, Arai S, Takeoka S, Ishiwata S, Suzuki M, Sato H (2016) Facilely fabricated luminescent nanoparticle Thermosensor for real-time microthermography in living animals. ACS Sensors 1:1222–1227. https://doi.org/10.1021/acssensors.6b00320
15. Childs PRN, Greenwood JR, Long CA (2000) Review of temperature measurement. Rev Sci Instrum 71:2959–2978. https://doi.org/10.1063/1.1305516
16. Wang C, Ruizhi Xu WT, Jiang X, Zhengyu Cui MW, Sun H, Kun Fang NG (2011) Determining intracellular temperature at single-cell level by a novel thermocouple method. Cell Res:1517–1519. https://doi.org/10.1038/cr.2011.117
17. Kim K, Chung J, Hwang G, Kwon O, Lee JS (2011) Quantitative measurement with scanning thermal microscope by preventing the distortion due to the heat transfer through the air. ACS Nano 5:8700–8709. https://doi.org/10.1021/nn2026325

18. Powe AM, Fletcher KA, St. Luce NN, Lowry M, Neal S, McCarroll ME, Oldham PB, McGown LB, Warner IM (2004) Molecular fluorescence, phosphorescence, and chemiluminescence spectrometry. Anal Chem 76:4614–4634. https://doi.org/10.1021/ac040095d
19. Jaque D, Vetrone F (2012) Luminescence nanothermometry. Nanoscale 4:4301–4326. https://doi.org/10.1039/c2nr30764b
20. Zhou J, del Rosal B, Jaque D, Uchiyama S, Jin D (2020) Advances and challenges for fluorescence nanothermometry. Nat Methods 17:967–980. https://doi.org/10.1038/s41592-020-0957-y
21. Gota C, Okabe K, Funatsu T, Harada Y, Uchiyama S (2009) Hydrophilic fluorescent nanogel thermometer for intracellular thermometry. J Am Chem Soc 131:2766–2767. https://doi.org/10.1021/ja807714j
22. Okabe K, Inada N, Gota C, Harada Y, Funatsu T, Uchiyama S (2012) Intracellular temperature mapping with a fluorescent polymeric thermometer and fluorescence lifetime imaging microscopy. Nat Commun 3:705. https://doi.org/10.1038/ncomms1714
23. Yang J-M, Yang H, Lin L (2011) Quantum dot nano thermometers reveal heterogeneous local thermogenesis in living cells. ACS Nano 5:5067–5071. https://doi.org/10.1021/nn201142f
24. Tanimoto R, Hiraiwa T, Nakai Y, Shindo Y, Oka K, Hiroi N, Funahashi A (2016) Detection of temperature difference in neuronal cells. Sci Rep 6:22071. https://doi.org/10.1038/srep22071
25. Francolon N, Boyer D, Leccia F, Jouberton E, Walter A, Bordeianu C, Parat A, Felder-Flesch D, Begin-Colin S, Miot-Noirault E et al (2016) Preparation of Core/Shell NaYF4:Yb, Tm@dendrons nanoparticles with enhanced Upconversion luminescence for in vivo imaging. Nanomed Nanotechnol Biol Med 12:2107–2113. https://doi.org/10.1016/j.nano.2016.05.020
26. Meijernik A, Blasse G, Sytsma J, de Mello Donega C, Ellens A (1996) Electron-phonon coupling in rare earth compounds. Acta Phys Pol A 90:109–119
27. Zhou J, Liu Q, Feng W, Sun Y, Li F (2015) Upconversion luminescent materials: advances and applications. Chem Rev 115:395–465. https://doi.org/10.1021/cr400478f
28. Vetrone F, Naccache R, Zamarrón A, Juarranz de la Fuente A, Sanz-Rodríguez F, Martinez Maestro L, Martín Rodriguez E, Jaque D, García Solé J, Capobianco JA (2010) Temperature sensing using fluorescent nanothermometers. ACS Nano 4:3254–3258. https://doi.org/10.1021/nn100244a
29. Vetrone F, Naccache R, Juarranz De La Fuente A, Sanz-Rodríguez F, Blazquez-Castro A, Rodriguez EM, Jaque D, Solé JG, Capobianco JA (2010) Intracellular imaging of HeLa cells by non-functionalized NaYF 4:Er3+, Yb3+ Upconverting nanoparticles. Nanoscale 2:495–498. https://doi.org/10.1039/b9nr00236g
30. Yang S-T, Cao L, Luo PG, Lu F, Wang X, Wang H, Meziani MJ, Liu Y, Qi G, Sun Y-P (2009) Carbon dots for optical imaging in vivo. J Am Chem Soc 131:11308–11309. https://doi.org/10.1021/ja904843x
31. Macairan J-R, Jaunky DB, Piekny A, Naccache R (2019) Intracellular ratiometric temperature sensing using fluorescent carbon dots. Nanoscale Adv 1. https://doi.org/10.1039/c8na00255j
32. Xie N, Huang J, Yang X, He X, Liu J, Huang J, Fang H (2017) Scallop-inspired DNA nanomachine : a ratiometric nanothermometer for intracellular temperature sensing. Anal Chem. https://doi.org/10.1021/acs.analchem.7b02709
33. Zhang H, Wu Y, Gan Z, Yang Y, Liu Y, Tang P, Wu D (2019) Accurate intracellular and: in vivo temperature sensing based on CuInS2/ZnS QD micelles. J Mater Chem B 7:2835–2844. https://doi.org/10.1039/c8tb03261k
34. Yang Y, Wu D (2020) Research shortcomings of fluorescent Nanothermometers in biological and medical fields. Nanomedicine 15:735–738. https://doi.org/10.2217/nnm-2019-0416
35. Shen Y, Santos HD, Ximendes E, Lifante J, Sanz-Portilla A, Monge L, Fernández N, Chaves-Coira I, Jacinto C, Brites C et al (2020) Ag2S nanoheaters with multiparameter sensing for reliable thermal feedback during in vivo tumor therapy. Adv Funct Mater 30. https://doi.org/10.1002/adfm.202002730

36. Ximendes EC, Rocha U, Del Rosal B, Vaquero A, Sanz-Rodríguez F, Monge L, Ren F, Vetrone F, Ma D, García-Solé J et al (2017) In vivo ischemia detection by luminescent nanothermometers. Adv Healthc Mater 6. https://doi.org/10.1002/adhm.201601195
37. Siesler, H.W. Vibrational spectroscopy; 2016; ISBN 9780128035818
38. Dutta A (2017) Fourier transform infrared spectroscopy. Elsevier Inc., Amsterdam; ISBN 9780323461405
39. Holton SE, Walsh MJ, Kajdacsy-Balla A, Bhargava R (2011) Label-free characterization of cancer-activated fibroblasts using infrared spectroscopic imaging. Biophys J 101:1513–1521. https://doi.org/10.1016/j.bpj.2011.07.055
40. Kumar S, Srinivasan A, Nikolajeff F (2017) Role of infrared spectroscopy and imaging in cancer diagnosis. Curr Med Chem 25:1055–1072. https://doi.org/10.2174/0929867324666170523121314
41. Gurion B, Sheva B, Sheva B (2004) Possible common biomarkers from FTIR microspectroscopy of. J Microsc 215:86–91
42. Lyng FM, Faoláin EÓ, Conroy J, Meade AD, Knief P, Duffy B, Hunter MB, Byrne JM, Kelehan P, Byrne HJ (2007) Vibrational spectroscopy for cervical cancer pathology, from biochemical analysis to diagnostic tool. Exp Mol Pathol 82:121–129. https://doi.org/10.1016/j.yexmp.2007.01.001
43. Antonacci, G. IR spectroscopic imaging for cancer diagnosis, 2010
44. Faoláin EÓ, Hunter MB, Byrne JM, Kelehan P, Byrne HJ, Lyng FM, Street K The potential of vibrational spectroscopy in the early detection of cervical cancer : an exciting Emerging Field Radiation and Environmental Science Centre (RESC), Focas Institute, Dublin Institute Of. 2005, 5826, 25–36, https://doi.org/10.1117/12.603344
45. Ali M. Raman Characterization of Structural Properties of Thermally Modified Nanographite
46. Kamemoto LE, Misra AK, Sharma SK, Goodman MT, Hugh LUK, Dykes AC, Acosta T (2010) Near-infrared micro-Raman spectroscopy for in vitro detection of cervical cancer. Appl Spectrosc 64:255–261. https://doi.org/10.1366/000370210790918364
47. Dacey GC, Ross IM (1955) The field effect transistor. Bell Syst Tech J 34:1149–1189. https://doi.org/10.1002/j.1538-7305.1955.tb03794.x
48. Schöning MJ, Poghossian A (2002) Recent advances in biologically sensitive field-effect transistors (BioFETs). Analyst 127:1137–1151. https://doi.org/10.1039/B204444G
49. Poghossian A, Yoshinobu T, Simonis A, Ecken H, Lüth H, Schöning MJ (2001) Penicillin detection by means of field-effect based sensors: EnFET, capacitive EIS sensor or LAPS? Sensors Actuators B Chem 78:237–242. https://doi.org/10.1016/S0925-4005(01)00819-X
50. Seo H-I, Kim C-S, Sohn B-K, Yeow T, Son M-T, Haskard M (1997) ISFET glucose sensor based on a new principle using the electrolysis of hydrogen peroxide. Sensors Actuators B Chem 40:1–5. https://doi.org/10.1016/S0925-4005(97)80191-8
51. Zhang A, Hou Y, Jaffrezic-Renault N, Wan J, Soldatkin A, Chovelon J-M (2002) Mixed urease/Amphiphile LB films and their application for biosensor development. Bioelectrochemistry 56:157–158. https://doi.org/10.1016/S1567-5394(02)00045-2
52. Bettaieb F, Ponsonnet L, Lejeune P, Ouada HB, Martelet C, Bakhrouf A, Jaffrézic-Renault N, Othmane A (2007) Immobilization of *E. Coli* bacteria in three-dimensional matrices for ISFET biosensor design. Bioelectrochemistry 71:118–125. https://doi.org/10.1016/j.bioelechem.2007.02.004
53. Xu J, Luo X, Chen H (2005) Analytical aspects of FET - based sensors. Anal Chem:420–430
54. Gopinath PG, Anitha VR, Mastani SA (2017) Design of Biosensor Array with current boost and signal conditioning circuits for HPV detection. Alexandria Eng J:1–11
55. Chen Y, Ren R, Pu H, Guo X, Chang J, Zhou G, Mao S, Kron M, Chen J (2017) Field-effect transistor biosensor for rapid detection of Ebola antigen. Sci Rep 7:10974. https://doi.org/10.1038/s41598-017-11387-7
56. Seo G, Lee G, Kim MJ, Baek S-H, Choi M, Ku KB, Lee C-S, Jun S, Park D, Kim HG et al (2020) Rapid detection of COVID-19 causative virus (SARS-CoV-2) in human nasopharyngeal

swab specimens using field-effect transistor-based biosensor. ACS Nano 14:5135–5142. https://doi.org/10.1021/acsnano.0c02823
57. Aspermair P, Mishyn V, Bintinger J, Happy H, Bagga K, Subramanian P, Knoll W, Boukherroub R, Szunerits S (2020) Reduced graphene oxide–based field effect transistors for the detection of E7 protein of human papillomavirus in saliva. Anal Bioanal Chem:7–11. https://doi.org/10.1007/s00216-020-02879-z
58. Braun T, Ghatkesar MK, Backmann N, Grange W, Boulanger P, Letellier L, Lang H, Bietsch A, Gerber C, Hegner M (2009) Membrane protein – ligand interactions using microcantilever Array sensors. Nat Nanotechnol 4:179–185. https://doi.org/10.1038/NNANO.2008.398
59. Arlett JL, Myers EB, Roukes ML (2011) Comparative advantages of mechanical biosensors. Nat Publ Gr 6:203–215. https://doi.org/10.1038/nnano.2011.44
60. Stylianou A (2018) AFM assessing of nanomechanical fingerprints for cancer early diagnosis and classification: from single cell to tissue level. Nanoscale:20930–20945. https://doi.org/10.1039/c8nr06146g
61. Kim N, Kim D, Cho Y (2009) Sensors and actuators B : chemical development of indirect-competitive quartz crystal microbalance immunosensor for C-reactive protein. Sensors Actuators B Chem 143:444–448. https://doi.org/10.1016/j.snb.2009.09.046
62. Yang LI, Huang X (2014) A novel piezoelectric immunosensor for early cervical cancer detection. In: Proceedings of the symposium on piezoelectricity, acoustic waves, and device applications, pp 453–456
63. Microbalance, Q.C.; At-cut, M.; Sauerbrey, T. QCM100- Quartz Crystal Microbalance Theory and Calibration The QCM oscillator. In; Vol. 9040
64. Osteryoung J (1771) Frequency of a quartz microbalance in contact with liquid. Anal Chem 1989:1770–1771
65. Dell D, Zavaglia M, Tombelli S, Bertacca G, Cavazzana AO, Bevilacqua G, Minunni M, Mascini M (2007) Development of combined DNA-based piezoelectric biosensors for the simultaneous detection and genotyping of high risk human papilloma virus strains. Clin Chim Acta 383:140–146. https://doi.org/10.1016/j.cca.2007.05.009
66. Jearanaikoon P, Prakrankamanant P, Leelayuwat C (2016) The evaluation of loop-mediated isothermal amplification-quartz crystal microbalance (LAMP-QCM) biosensor as a real-time measurement of HPV16 DNA. J Virol Methods 229:8–11. https://doi.org/10.1016/j.jviromet.2015.12.005
67. Notomi T, Okayama H, Masubuchi H, Yonekawa T, Watanabe K, Amino N, Hase T (2000) Loop-mediated isothermal amplification of DNA. Nucleic Acids Res 28
68. White RM, Voltmer FW (1965) Direct piezoelectric coupling to surface elastic waves. Appl Phys Lett 314:10–13. https://doi.org/10.1063/1.1754276
69. Länge K, Rapp BE, Rapp M (2008) Surface acoustic wave biosensors : a review. Anal Bioanal Chem:1509–1519. https://doi.org/10.1007/s00216-008-1911-5
70. Mahle N, Pfeiffer C, Parker W (1979) Surface acoustic wave probe for chemical analysis. Anal Chem 51:1458–1464
71. Eh E, Sciences M (2011) Streaming by leaky surface acoustic waves. Proc Royal Soc A Mathematical Phys Eng Sci:1779–1800
72. Wang Y, Chen M, Zhang L, Ding Y, Luo Y, Xu Q, Shi J, Cao L, Fu W (2009) Rapid detection of human papilloma virus using a novel leaky surface acoustic wave peptide nucleic acid biosensor. Biosens Bioelectron 24:3455–3460. https://doi.org/10.1016/j.bios.2009.04.034
73. Gao S, Wang X (2011) Microelectromechanical system-based diagnostic technology for cervical cancer. J Cancer Res Clin Oncol:1721–1727. https://doi.org/10.1007/s00432-011-1019-8
74. Prakash P, Patne SCU, Singh AK, Kumar M, Mishra MN, Gulati AK (2016) PCR and genotyping for HPV in cervical cancer patients. J Glob Infect Dis 8:100–107. https://doi.org/10.4103/0974-777X.188591
75. Elnifro EM, Ashshi AM, Cooper RJ (2000) Multiplex PCR : optimization and application in diagnostic virology. Clin Microbiol Rev 13:559–570

76. Surriabre P, Torrico A, Vargas T, Ugarte F, Rodriguez P (2019) Assessment of a new low-cost, PCR-based strategy for high-risk human papillomavirus DNA detection for cervical cancer prevention. BMC Infect Dis:1–7
77. Kim SJ, Nahm KB, Lim JB, Oh SW, Choi EY (2014) A rapid and sensitive detection of HPV by combined assay of PCR and fluorescence DNA Chip. Biochip J 8:48–54. https://doi.org/10.1007/s13206-014-8108-0
78. Xu Y, Liu Y, Wu Y, Xia X, Liao Y, Li Q (2014) Fluorescent probe-based lateral flow assay for multiplex nucleic acid detection. Anal Chem:5611–5614. https://doi.org/10.1021/ac5010458
79. Pierce KE, Sanchez JA, Rice JE, Wangh LJ (2005) Linear-after-the-exponential (LATE) -PCR : primer design criteria for high yields of specific single- stranded DNA and improved real-time detection. PNAS 102:8609–8614
80. Wang CC (2020) An optical biosensors: an exhaustive and comprehensive review. RSC Anal. https://doi.org/10.4103/0974-777X.188591
81. Strianese M, Staiano M, Ruggiero G, Labella T, Pellecchia C, Auria SD Fluorescence-Based Biosensors. *875*, https://doi.org/10.1007/978-1-61779-806-1
82. Mawatari K, Sato K, Tanaka Y (2010) Microbead-based rolling circle amplification in a microchip for sensitive DNA detection. Lab Chip:1262–1266. https://doi.org/10.1039/b927460j
83. Zhang H, Liu L, Li C, Fu H, Chen Y, Yang M (2011) Multienzyme-nanoparticles amplification for sensitive virus genotyping in microfluidic microbeads Array using au nanoparticle probes and quantum dots as labels. Biosens Bioelectron 29:89–96. https://doi.org/10.1016/j.bios.2011.07.074
84. Yue W, Zou H, Jin Q, Li C, Xu T, Fu H (2014) Single layer linear array of microbeads for multiplexed analysis of DNA and proteins. Biosens Bioelectron 54:297–305. https://doi.org/10.1016/j.bios.2013.10.034
85. Baek TJ, Park PY, Han KN (2008) Development of a photodiode Array biochip using a bipolar semiconductor and its application to detection of human papilloma virus. Anal Bioanal Chem:1373–1378. https://doi.org/10.1007/s00216-007-1814-x

FSC
www.fsc.org
MIX
Papier | Fördert gute Waldnutzung
FSC® C083411

Kolibri 360 GmbH
Ferdinand-Jühlke-Straße 7
99095 Erfurt, Deutschland
produktsicherheit@kolibri360.de